Praise from friends of Jim Tietjens

"Jim is a true friend, like a brother. He's always been there for me. He inspires, he pushes, he supports, and he never judges….no matter what." — **Dominic Barczewski**, high school teammate, professional soccer player, St. Louis Soccer Hall of Fame

"Jim was an incredible athlete in his younger days. I believe it was the attention to his everyday fitness regimen that enabled him to persevere through hereditary issues early on. Jim's continued fitness, post-playing days, allowed him to recover from numerous transplants that followed. He is a fighter and a survivor." — **Bill Colletta**, high school teammate

"When I think of Jim Tietjens, I see a man who has guts and determination. Through his soccer playing career he showed a desire and dedication to be the best, not ever giving up, and he carries this through his life filled with many health setbacks. Jim had to endure two heart transplants, cancer and many other issues in recovery. This took courage, perseverance and determination to beat all odds to be there for his family and friends. Every time I speak with Jim, it is not about himself, but about others. He always asks how I am doing and other friends' health, willing to spend time with others to help them recuperate. I respect Jim so much for the man he is." — **Larry Hulcer**, former teammate, professional soccer player, St. Louis Soccer Hall of Fame

"When I think of Jim, I am in awe of how he has carried himself throughout his life's highest and lowest points. As an Olympian and professional soccer player, Jim has always remained humble and has never allowed himself to be defined by his achievements. He has always been thoughtful, kind and willing to give advice to help fellow teammates reach their own personal goals and aspirations." — **Perry Van Der Beck**, former teammate, professional soccer player, St. Louis Soccer Hall of Fame

"I have known Tietj since I was 3 years old, and I cannot think of a more resilient, gritty character that I have come across in my 56 years of knowing him. He is a living lesson in perseverance." — **Mike McCartney**, childhood friend, Indiana University soccer alum

"Jim Tietjens is simply one of the hardest working, most determined people you will ever meet. Transitioning from a highly successful professional soccer player to an accomplished business career at Rawlings and Anheuser-Busch while overcoming the challenges of two heart and a kidney transplant along with fighting cancer…and you name it. Jim is a testament of an unparalleled fighter and an inspiration to anyone who has had the privilege to know him." — **Mike Redohl**, childhood friend

"When I hear the name Jim Tietjens the first thing that comes to my mind is he is a winner. He is a special person with a heart of gold. He is someone you can always count on and is always looking to help others. He is disciplined, strong, a fighter, caring and someone I'm privileged to call my friend and teammate." — **Johnny Hayes**, former teammate, professional soccer player, St. Louis Soccer Hall of Fame

"Jim has always demanded the best of himself. Roadblocks are simply challenges to overcome. Most could not have overcome the major issues that Jim has had to endure. Two heart transplants, a kidney transplant, Non Hodgkin's Lymphoma, tongue and throat cancer and three years of dialysis. Jim never asked to come out of the game. As he did on the field, he was determined to go the full 90. The fear, sorrow, despair, uncertainty, tears and loneliness — they have finally come to an end. His heart will live on forever in this life and the next, in the young and old who have witnessed his journey of courage and love. His story stands the test of time."
— **Gary Ullo**, high school teammate

SAVES

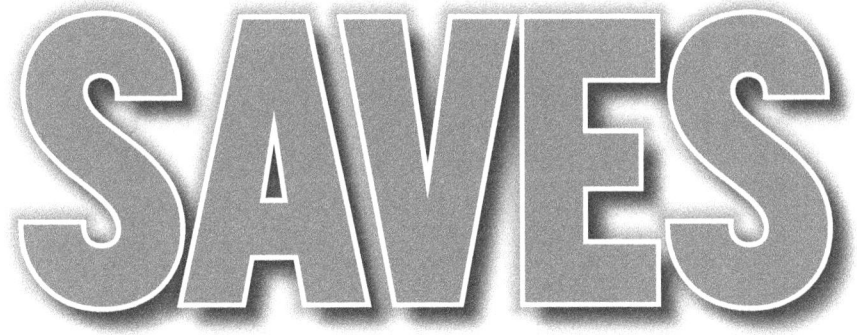

SAVES

The Amazing Story of American Goalkeeper Jim Tietjens

with Jeff Kuchno

InspireMe Stories Publishing

Dedication

To my mother.
Mom knew the challenges I would face in my life and from a very young age took my hand and taught me to be brave and never back down.

My sisters Karen and Laura.
Both fought two very different battles.
They accepted their health challenges with bravery, grace and peace.

Jimmy, Annie and Julie.
You were always the "wind beneath my wings" and my love for the three of you always slanted the odds in my favor.

To my entire medical family at Barnes Hospital.

To my brothers, and you all know who you are.

To Craig Reiss and Cindy Pasque.
What you did to save my life and allow me to be a father and a husband. Such a gift that God brought you into my life.

To both my donors... one I never knew of... and Colton, who I've learned so much about.

And finally my father Jim. I hope I have made you proud, pops.

SAVES

The Amazing Story of American Goalkeeper Jim Tietjens
Jim Tietjens with Jeff Kuchno

Published by InspireMe Stories Publishing, LLC,
Copyright ©2024 Jim Tietjens and Jeff Kuchno, InspireMe Stories Publishing, LLC
All rights reserved.

No part of this publication may be reproduced, stored in a retrieval system, or transmitted in any form or by any means, electronic, mechanical, photocopying, recording, scanning, or otherwise, except as permitted under Section 107 or 108 of the 1976 United States Copyright Act, without the prior written permission of the Publisher. Requests to the Publisher for permission should be addressed to Permissions Department, InspireMe Stories Publishing, LLC, inspiremestoriespublishing@gmail.com.

Limit of Liability/Disclaimer of Warranty: While the publisher and author have used their best efforts in preparing this book, they make no representations or warranties with respect to the accuracy or completeness of the contents of this book and specifically disclaim any implied warranties of merchantability or fitness for a particular purpose. No warranty may be created or extended by sales representatives or written sales materials. The advice and strategies contained herein may not be suitable for your situation. You should consult with a professional where appropriate. Neither the publisher nor author shall be liable for any loss of profit or any other commercial damages, including but not limited to special, incidental, consequential, or other damages.

Project Management and Book Design: DavisCreativePublishing.com

Names: Tietjens, Jim, author. | Kuchno, Jeff, author.
Title: Saves : the amazing story of American goalkeeper Jim Tietjens / [Jim Tietjens], with Jeff Kuchno.
Description: St. Louis, MO : InspireMe Stories Publishing, [2024]
Identifiers: ISBN: 979-8-9898929-0-7 (paperback) | 979-8-9898929-2-1 (hardback) | 979-8-9898929-1-4 (ebook) | LCCN: 2024901273
Subjects: LCSH: Tietjens, Jim. | Soccer players--Missouri--Saint Louis--Biography. | Soccer goalkeepers--Missouri--Saint Louis--Biography. | Heart--Transplantation--Patients-- Biography. | Cancer--Patients--Biography. | LCGFT: Autobiographies. | BISAC: MEDICAL / Surgery / Transplant. | HEALTH & FITNESS / Diseases & Conditions / Heart. | SPORTS & RECREATION / Soccer.
Classification: LCC: GV942.7.T525 A3 2024 | DDC: 796.334092--dc23

ATTENTION CORPORATIONS, UNIVERSITIES, COLLEGES AND PROFESSIONAL ORGANIZATIONS: Quantity discounts are available on bulk purchases of this book for educational, gift purposes, or as premiums for increasing magazine subscriptions or renewals. Special books or book excerpts can also be created to fit specific needs. For information, please contact InspireMe Stories Publishing, LLC, inspiremestoriespublishing@gmail.com.

Table of Contents

	Foreword xi
	Introduction. xv
Chapter 1	Growing Up in South County .1
Chapter 2	High School Success 9
Chapter 3	International Soccer 17
Chapter 4	Choosing St. Louis U. 25
Chapter 5	Playing Pro Soccer 31
Chapter 6	Caravan Man 41
Chapter 7	Karen's Death 45
Chapter 8	Julie 49
Chapter 9	Slowing Down 51
Chapter 10	First Transplant 59
Chapter 11	Back To Work 63
Chapter 12	The Kids 65
Chapter 13	McGwire Mania. 71
Chapter 14	My Dream Job 75
Chapter 15	Cancer 79
Chapter 16	Marital Trouble 83
Chapter 17	A Difficult Summer. 87
Chapter 18	Meeting My Donor's Family 93
Chapter 19	Mid-America Transplant 99
Chapter 20	Pneumonia. 103
Chapter 21	My Oakville Brothers 107
Chapter 22	Peripheral Artery Disease 113
Chapter 23	Hall of Fame 115
Chapter 24	My Sister Laura 119
Chapter 25	Thanks / Acknowledgments 121
	More praise for Jim Tietjens 127
	Foundation to Advance Vascular Cures. 133
	About the Authors. 137

Foreword

I met Jim Tietjens at the 1975 Oakville High School boys fall soccer tryouts. It was immediately evident that he possessed great athletic ability and a tremendous thirst for knowledge. He always looked for ways to improve his goalkeeper skills.

Out of the seven goalies attending the 1975 tryouts, Jim, a sophomore, was selected as the No. 1 starting goalkeeper over the six upperclassmen because he had the "whole package." Jim possessed great athletic ability, quick decision-making skills, agility, and reliable hands, plus he was a hard worker who trained as intensely as many college and professional goalies.

Jim continued to improve his goalkeeper skills during the next nine months in preparation for the 1976 fall season. He led the Oakville Tigers, who were not included in the preseason rankings, to a very successful regular season record. During the 1976 playoffs, Jim started to dominate games against highly ranked private schools, leading the Tigers to several upset victories on their way to the 1976 Missouri state high school championship match. Many spectators who attended this state final game, including opposing players and coaches, speak about Jim's play on that day as the greatest performance ever by a Missouri high school goalie. He led the Oakville Tigers to a 1-0 victory, making numerous phenomenal saves and fearlessly coming out of his goal to intercept dangerous high balls that were sent into his penalty area. Every spectacular save not only demoralized the opposition little by little, but also inspired his teammates and led the squad to an amazing victory.

As a result of Jim's tremendous ability, he was selected as a member of the U.S. Youth National soccer team. What a well-deserved fantastic opportunity. Jim missed the majority of the 1977 high school season and upon his return the high school playoffs were ready to begin. A decision was made to start the goalkeeper who had played in all of the games during the regular season. Jim not only unselfishly supported his fellow goalkeeper, he also advised and helped prepare him for these important matches. Jim's unselfishness sent an important inspirational message to the entire team.

I was so excited and proud that Jim was offered and accepted a soccer scholarship to attend Saint Louis University, my alma mater. As a sign of my excitement and appreciation, I gifted Jim one of my three NCAA championship coats. It was a pleasure watching Jim earn the starting keeper position with SLU for the next two seasons before he moved on, signing a professional contract with the Fort Lauderdale Strikers of the North American Soccer League.

Jim utilized these same qualities, learned as an athlete, during his subsequent years when he faced numerous health challenges — "working hard, making tough decisions during difficult times, and fearlessly doing whatever was needed to get the job done."

Tietj was an inspiration to many individuals who had serious heart issues, including my wife. They were both in attendance at a 1994 American Heart Association charity event. Jim received his first heart transplant in 1992. My wife was a two-year starter with the Washington University women's soccer team. However, in 1993, she underwent open heart surgery to repair a hole in her heart and was experiencing a very difficult recovery. She spoke with Jim at the AHA event and remembers him as an extremely kind, caring and supportive individual. Being a fellow soccer player who had a successful heart transplant, Jim provided hope and inspiration during her long, difficult recovery period. Both had the same attitude — "I'm an athlete. I will overcome any obstacle or challenge that is thrown at me."

Many athletes, especially in team sports like soccer, develop permanent bonds with their teammates. This is definitely the case with Jim, who has remained extremely close to many of his high school, college, and professional teammates — "brothers for life" who over the years have celebrated together and have supported each other during good times and bad.

Personally, I feel blessed that I met Jim Tietjens when he was a 15-year old kid and that we have remained friends and confidants over the years. Life is short. Cherish your family, friends and "brothers."
— **Jim Bokern**

Note: Jim Bokern coached at Oakville High School in St. Louis from 1975 to 1978. He guided Oakville to the state championship in 1976 and was named the Missouri High School Soccer Coach of the Year. As a player, he was a member of three national championship teams at St. Louis University. He then played three seasons of professional soccer for the St. Louis Stars of the North American Soccer League. During his career as a player and coach, he was part of 11 national championship teams and three high school champions. He was inducted into the St. Louis Soccer Hall of Fame in 2005.

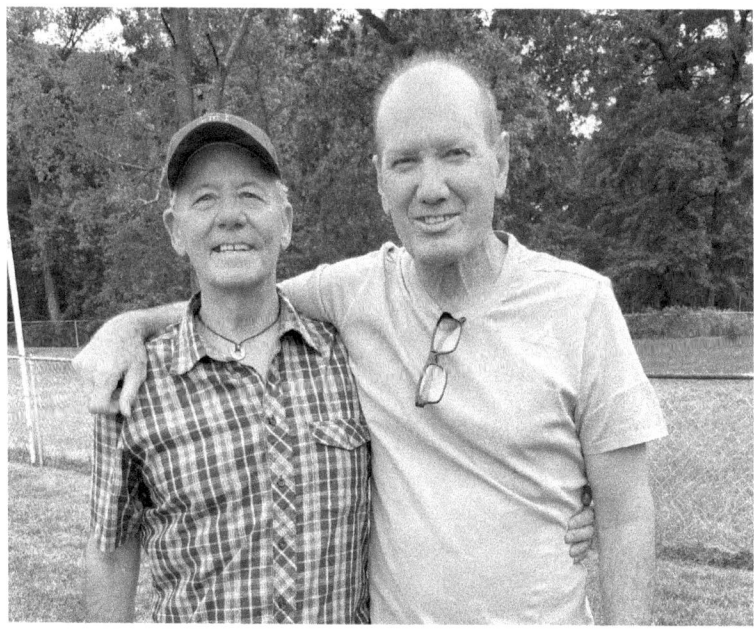

Jim with Jim Bokern

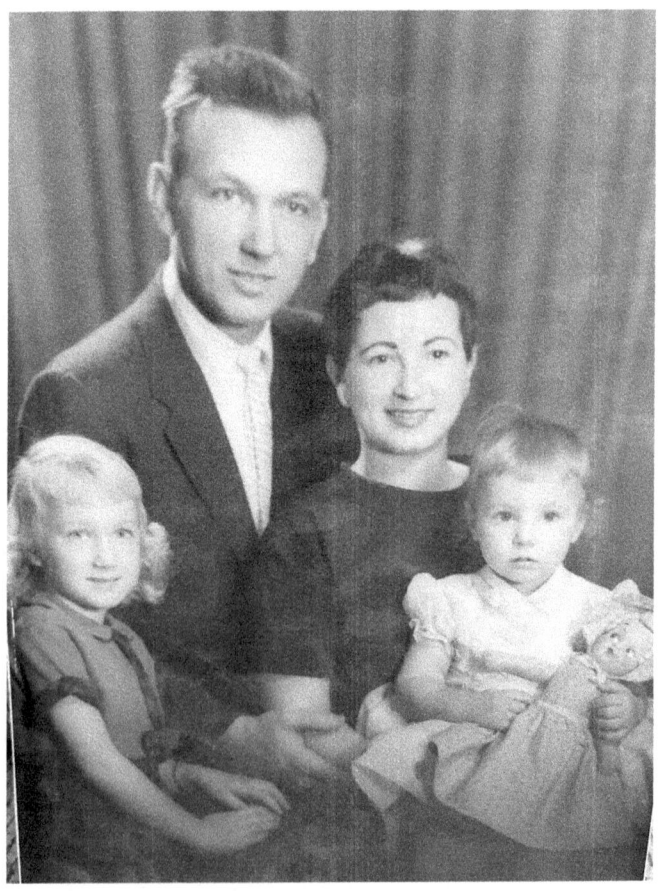

Jim's dad, mom, sisters Laura and Karen, circa 1959

Introduction

My dad was a good athlete. Tall and thin, he swam, played football and basketball, and ran track in school. He was also an avid fisherman and a duck hunter who enjoyed camping, a guy who just loved the outdoors.

At least that's what I have been told.

I really don't have any memories of my dad. James Arthur Tietjens (*pronounced TEE-jenz*) passed away in November 1961 when I was less than two years old. He died at the young age of 32 from a heart condition known as myocarditis, an inflammation of the heart muscle that reduces the ability of the heart to pump blood (*the term for this disease today is idiopathic cardiomyopathy*). It's an illness I didn't know much about as a young boy growing up in South St. Louis County.

My dad was an accomplished college athlete. He played college football at the Missouri School of Mines in Rolla (*now Missouri University of Science and Technology*) from 1948 to 1951. As a senior, he led the Miners in pass receptions and receiving yards. After that season, he was named a first team all-conference tight end. He also was a member of the school's track team.

Like my dad, I played all kinds of sports as a kid. (*I also loved to go fishing… I guess I got that from him, too*). I started playing organized sports when I got into grade school, mainly baseball and soccer. By the time I got to high school, I realized that soccer was the sport for me.

As a junior in high school, I helped my team win the state soccer championship in 1976. My success as the goalkeeper on that team led to an opportunity to represent my country as a member of the United States youth national team. We traveled the world playing in other countries — Holland, Italy, Switzerland, France, Germany, Honduras, you name it. After high school, I played two seasons of college soccer at St. Louis University before beginning a professional career that lasted five seasons. For a while, soccer was my life.

And then it wasn't.

Injuries — I had three knee surgeries by age 26 — ended my soccer career. I also inherited the gene that causes cardiomyopathy from my dad, and that almost ended my life.

I knew something was wrong when my sister Karen became sick from the same "bad" heart gene. She died of this heart illness in 1989 when I was 29 years old; she was 32. It was around this time that I started slowing down physically. I, too, had the same "bad" heart gene. Three years later, I had a heart transplant that saved my life. However, this was the beginning of a lifetime of health challenges for me.

Starting with my first operation, I have had two heart transplants and one kidney transplant. I have had cancer twice. I have had pneumonia at least 12 times. I have been dealing with circulation problems that led to the amputation of one of my toes. I can't remember many times during the last 30 years when I have not had a major health challenge to overcome.

However, while I spent most of my athletic career making saves on the soccer field, my adult life has been blessed with wonderful friends, family, doctors and nurses who have saved me over and over. I've had a lot of suffering in my life, but God has given me the strength to endure that suffering. He has given me special friends to support me. He has given me some of the greatest medical people in the world. My suffering has put wonderful people in my life. I have had so much support, there's no way I could have done this by myself.

This book is about more than personal perseverance and accomplishments. It's about the power of family, faith and friends. It's a story of "Saves."

Chapter 1

Growing Up in South County

Most people feel they have the greatest mom in the world, but that's how I felt — I had the greatest mom in the world. I saw how my mom lived, how strong she was. Three kids under the age of 7, losing a husband at age 32, and seeing that we never suffered. We played sports, we had clothes, we had food. Just by watching her, my mom taught me that we can overcome anything. That belief has always been with me.

When I was 6, my mom got remarried to a man by the name of Harold Richter. Harold's wife had passed away from cancer during their first year of marriage. I never had a real father-son relationship with Harold, but I gave him a lot of credit for coming into a family with three small children and taking us on. I had a lot of respect for the man.

My mom and Harold had two children together — my half-brother Bill and my half-sister Chrissy. I remember when my brother Bill was born. I remember coming home from school (*I think I was in fourth grade*), running straight into the house, and going to the crib to see this amazing baby in my life. A few years later — when I was 12 — Chrissy was born.

A Sports Fanatic

From a very young age, I was always interested in sports. My sisters played softball (*in fact, mom tried to coach their team, even though she wasn't very athletic*), I would see them play, and from kindergarten on I wanted to have a baseball or football in my hand. It really wasn't a soccer ball until we moved close to St. Margaret Mary Alacoque Catholic Parish in Oakville.

No matter what it was in the neighborhood, we were always playing sports. Many times it was street hockey — remember, the St. Louis Blues were an expansion team in 1967 — and we even played a little ice hockey in the winter. I loved hockey, loved soccer, loved baseball. Like all kids at that time, we would ride on our bikes in the summer. We would have our ball glove hanging from the handle bar and we'd have our bat. We would leave in the morning and come home dusty in the evening from playing baseball all day. We would play soccer in the backyards of friends. It was a great time.

My mother — as I mentioned — was not athletic. But she WAS a good bowler. She and some of the other mothers from the subdivision had a team that bowled at what is now DuBowl Lanes on Lemay Ferry. They were very competitive. My mom was competitive. She did not like to lose.

One year my mom's team lost the league championship by one pin. They thought there might have been a mistake in the score of the game, so that night Billy Schornheuser (*his mom was on the team*) and I went up to the bowling alley and we went through the trash cans looking for the scoresheets to see if we could find the

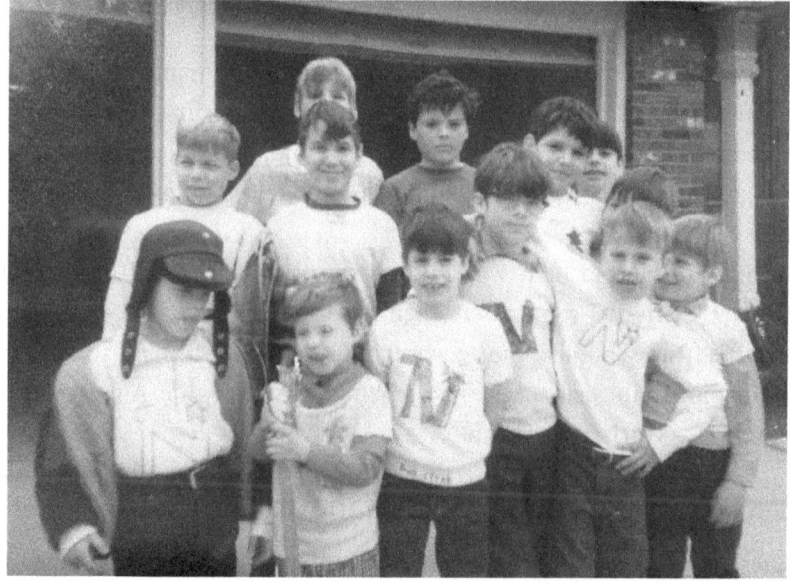

The kids in the neighborhood

mistake. Three of the moms were with us with flashlights. We were physically in the dumpsters sloshing through everything — half-eaten burgers, fries, drinks. There were tons of scoresheets in there, but we could not find the one from that day. We went through everything. It was sickening.

The most exciting thing, though, was when I saw my mom bowl a 270 game. I was at the bowling alley and she asked me to go to the stand and get her a hamburger. I did, and I put an X on her burger with ketchup (*because that's the mark for a strike*). Through eight frames, she was perfect. In those days, they would make announcements before a game was even over. "JoAnn Richter is on Lane 8 rolling a perfect game," the voice said. My mom was all pissed off about that, and she ended up rolling a 270. But I was so proud when I heard my mom's name on the intercom. "That's so huge," I thought.

My Best Friend Mike

It was soon after we moved to Oakville that I became friends with Mike Redohl. In fact, we are still best friends today. We grew up in the same subdivision. We had a lot of young families in the neighborhood. He grew up on the street opposite from our house, and his house was the center of activity in the neighborhood.

We played everything — Indian Ball, football, basketball, hockey. I was barred from playing hockey by my step-dad (*I lost a tooth once playing hockey*), but I could play over there. Their garage door took a beating, but his parents didn't mind. As long as we were active and staying busy, they were happy.

About the tooth, there's a funny story. I lost my tooth on Super Bowl Sunday in '69 (*when Joe Namath led the Jets to an upset victory over the Colts*). It was down the street where they were building new homes. Water had gathered from rains and had frozen over. It was a big enough area to skate on. I was over there with a few guys and then there was Sharon Ladd, this girl I was in love with as a kid. For some reason, she had a hockey stick. I was skating past her with my head down and her stick came up and hit me in the mouth. It broke off half of my tooth.

I had to go home and was essentially barred forever from playing hockey, but we always played hockey in front of Redohl's house. Harold never went to any street other than ours, so he didn't know. He did say, though, that I wouldn't have lost my tooth if I had stayed home and watched the Super Bowl.

South County Soccer Champs

It was at St. Margaret Mary where I first played organized sports. I was signed up to play soccer. My mom did that because everyone else was doing it. I remember my first pair of soccer shoes — high-top Converse tennis shoes — that were split in the front. My step-dad took duct tape and put it around the shoe so I could play. Later they bought me my first pair of "real" soccer shoes. They were GOLA soccer shoes that were two sizes too big because they had to fit me for a while. We had to stuff newspaper in the end of the shoe so my foot was not flapping around inside there.

We had a really good team at St. Margaret Mary. We played pretty much with the same guys year after year. Our coach, Mr. Fitzgerald, put me in goal because I was sort of big for my age and had good hand-eye

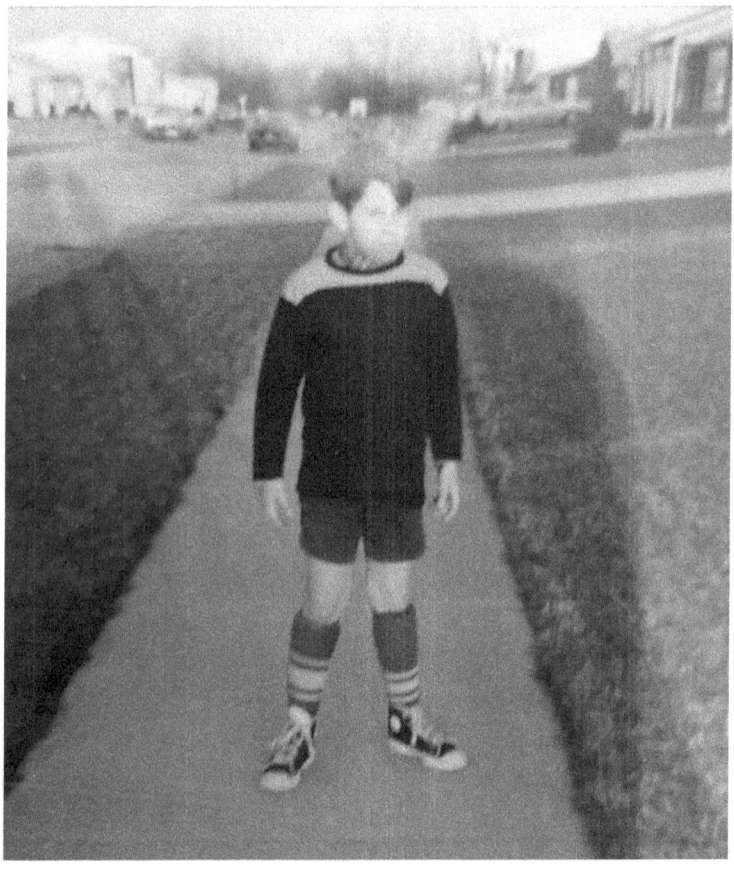

Jim in first grade

coordination. I even had my own jersey that I brought from home. It was a long-sleeve shirt that was black and had gold rings around the arms. Even in first grade, I was into what I was wearing. I stayed as the goalkeeper for eight years. We won our division eight straight years and won multiple South County championships.

I remember playing in a championship game at St. Francis of Assisi when I had the flu. I had a really high temperature, 101 or 102. Mr. Fitz told my mom, "Mrs. Richter, we have to have Jim, we have to have Jim for the game." I remember going out there on a cold day wearing a sweatsuit, pair of shorts, hat, gloves. I didn't go to warm up or anything. I was sitting under the pavilion at St. Francis and right when they were getting ready to kick off, I took my jacket off and ran down to the field. I did the same thing at halftime. I had a blanket on me during halftime and then went down to the field for the second half. We won the game, even though I felt horrible.

I also remember playing in the cold one year against St. Justin in the South County championship. We were playing at Bohrer Park in South County, and it was freezing. The parents were watching the game from their cars. I remember making a save, catching the ball as it was rolling toward our net, and all the horns are going off in the cars. That was their way of cheering for me. You're a young kid and it made you feel pretty good.

Mr. Fitz kept me in goal because he knew we needed a good foundation, and I was decent. But I always wanted to play out in the field and he would allow me to do that very few times. I remember one time playing out in the field I got the ball in front of my own goal and I dribbled all the way down the field and didn't even shoot. I just dribbled around the goalie and dribbled the ball into the goal. That's not good for the other team, you know, to make them look bad. It's not something you should do.

Another time Mr. Fitz allowed me to take a penalty kick. I was lined up to take the kick, but as I ran up to the ball I hit my toe on the ground first and the ball just dribbled into the goalie's hands. It was the most embarrassing moment I've ever had on the soccer field. I had to run all the way back to my goal. Suffice to say, Mr. Fitz never let me take another penalty kick.

Hard Work Pays Off

I always felt that I could outwork people at my level. I thought I was a good athlete; I never thought I was a great athlete. As a kid, I always believed in hard work. I would shovel driveways in the winter, sell tomatoes in the summer, sell newspapers

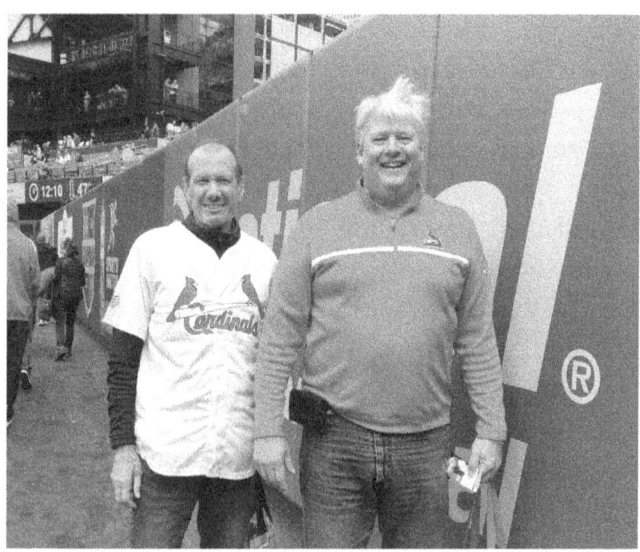

Jim with Mike Redohl

in front of Central Hardware. And I worked about 40 hours a week during the summer as a janitor at St. Margaret Mary. I was always trying to make money.

Having money in my pocket allowed me to do some fun things. Mike and I were Cardinals baseball fanatics. We would get on a bus and take that to Red Bird Lanes in South St. Louis, where we would catch another bus that would take us to Busch Stadium. We probably went to about 25 to 35 games a summer.

Sometimes when there was an afternoon game, we would leave around 9:30, 10 o'clock in the morning because we wanted to get to the ballpark early. We would stay after the games and wait for the teams to come out. One time against Atlanta the Braves came out to get on their bus and Hank Aaron threw me a baseball out of the bus window.

There was another time, though, when we didn't stick around after a game. Mike, who was 16 and just started driving, drove us downtown on this night in his dad's blue Regal. The Cardinals were losing big. I told Mike, "let's go, let's beat the traffic." He would say, "no, let's wait." I said, "no, we're leaving."

So we left early. As we listened on Mike's car radio, the Cardinals started coming back. Every time the Cardinals would get a hit, Mike was just screaming, "Aw, we should have stayed." By the time we got home, the Cardinals were on their way to scoring in the 12th inning to win the game, 10-9. I told Mike "we can't go in the house because Harold's going to know we left early. He's going to ask us about the game." So we just stayed outside and sat in the driveway because the game was just ending.

We messed that one up, but we had a great time going to the Cardinals games. We really enjoyed ourselves.

Mike's Dad

I also enjoyed getting to know Mike's dad, "Mick." His dad was always doing group stuff with the kids in the neighborhood. He was an interesting guy. He served as a captain in the U.S. Army. He paid his own way to the University of Notre Dame. And then he started his own business — the American Association of Industrial Management. It was a very successful consulting company. He would meet with some of the top business leaders around St. Louis.

Mike's dad was also the head of the Notre Dame alumni club in St. Louis. He would get all the guest speakers for their events. I remember one time when I was 15 and Mike was 16, we drove to the airport to pick up Digger Phelps, the famous Notre Dame basketball coach. We went straight to the gate to pick him up. He was wearing a powder blue leisure suit with a carnation on his lapel. He had a really cool navy blue leather suit bag with an Irish ND on the bag, a gold "Digger" embroidered above the ND. I carried that to the car and we had a great conversation with him. He talked about his team and how successful they were. He was very engaging.

We took Digger to the Missouri Athletic Club, where he gave a great talk. They had a raffle at the event and I won a Notre Dame t-shirt. It was sort of a gray workout shirt with a navy blue ND on it. I wore that thing for years. I just loved it. For a kid never winning anything in my life, it was cool.

Although I spent a lot of time with Mike Redohl, there were other guys in the neighborhood that became good friends. A lot of my friends, including Mike, went to Vianney (*high school*). We didn't have the funds, so it was never an option for me. But I was fine with going to Oakville. I grew up in Oakville. It was right down the road. I felt like it was the school I was supposed to attend.

Chapter 2

High School Success

When I started my freshman year at Oakville, I decided I didn't want to play goalie on the soccer team. I had this illusion I could be a field player. I was decent in the field, but not that good. I thought I would play on the freshman team and just have some fun.

I also played football as a freshman (*remember, high school soccer back then was played in the winter; it became a fall season sport my sophomore year*). I noticed how football attracted the ladies, so I tried it. I played tight end. I had good hands. It was cool, but I knew it wasn't my calling.

My sophomore year I started the soccer season on the B team. But it became apparent that the varsity was looking for a goalie. They had three other goalies at the start of the season, but there were some injuries and they needed someone. Some of the guys on varsity knew I was a goalie. They kept telling the coach to bring me up.

Jim Bokern, the varsity coach, called me into his office one day and said, "I'm hearing you can play goalie. We could really use one." I was excited for the opportunity. "I would love to be a part of it," I said.

Making My Mark On Varsity

So I moved up to varsity as a sophomore. Jim's brother, Dan Bokern, came out to our practices about three times a week. We would go on our own and he would shoot on me. Not many players could hit a ball as hard as he could. He would be pounding on me. He gave me the confidence that not many people could beat me.

I really worked on the technical part of the game. I started to watch a lot of German soccer on TV — *Soccer Made in Germany* — and studied the goalies. Sepp Maier was my idol in those days. He was the goalie on Germany's national team. Very flamboyant. A top goalie in the world. *Soccer Made in Germany* would be on TV Thursday nights and then they would show it again Sunday mornings. Even if they showed the same game, I would watch it because I was so focused on watching Sepp Maier and learning from him.

The German goalies were usually very big, they wore oversized gloves, and they pranced around the goal. When a player was getting ready to shoot, they would do a little hop step as a jump to get out and cut down the angle. I really modeled myself after them. I wasn't as tall as other goalies (*about 5-foot-11 at the time*), so I had to challenge shooters to cut down the angle.

I also brought some of the German style to St. Louis. The German goalies wore long shorts, baggy shirts, socks pulled up to the knees. I just thought it was the coolest thing in the world, so I would take my sweatpants and cut them off just above the knees. We were also able to order the goalie jerseys from Germany. They were advertised on *Soccer Made in Germany* and you could order a catalog or call a 1-800 number. Sepp Maier always wore blue with a black collar and black trim on the sleeves of his shirt. I would order one of those and I remember when they would come in the mail. Man, that was sweet.

By the middle of my sophomore season, I was starting almost every game. I had really good communication with my backs. I knew everyone's strengths. It was a great union. We won 15 games that year, 13 of them shutouts. My confidence was growing as a goalkeeper. I knew I could play at this level.

I also received help from family and friends. I don't think my mom ever missed one of my games. And Mike Redohl, he came to pretty much every game I played in high school. I would come home after a game, eat dinner, then walk to Mike's house so we could talk about the game.

We had some good players on my first varsity team. Gary Ullo, who became one of my best friends, was one of several all-conference players. John Gorman and Greg Hartmann were all-state defenders. Dominic Barczewski and Bill Colletta rounded out the backfield. When I got in there with that crew, I just felt so comfortable. It really made my job easy. They trusted me, I trusted them. There was no concern about having a sophomore goalie on the varsity.

We lost to Vianney in districts my sophomore year. We lost on a penalty kick. I came close to stopping it and didn't get it. But that season was a turning point for me. I was the last guy to ask a girl out to a dance, but I was confident on the field. I could see other goalies on the teams we played. I knew I was better.

After my sophomore year, I played club ball for South County Dutch in the Pepsi League. I remember signing up for a spot with the club team. We had a meeting in the gym at St. George Elementary School and Freddy Vasquez, who played on the 1964 U.S. Olympic team, was the trainer. He asked me what position I play. Without thinking, I told him midfielder. He said, "We don't need midfielders."

So, I'm walking out the door and Mr. Ullo (*Gary's dad*) stops me. "Where the hell are you going?" he yelled. I said, "They don't need me. I told them I'm a midfielder." "What the hell do you think you're doing?" he shouted back at me. "Get the hell back in there."

He walked me back to the table and told Freddy, "This is your goalie." So they signed me up to be their goalkeeper. If he had not done that, maybe I never would have achieved the things I did in soccer.

We had a great club team. We were coached by Don Bayer. He was best known for his coaching success at St. Francis and later he went into the St. Louis Soccer Hall of Fame. We beat a lot of good teams. We lost to Imo's Pizza in the National Cup Tournament. They beat us in a game at Forest Park and went on to win the National Junior Cup.

But my confidence as a goalkeeper continued to grow. Forget the nonsense about being a field player. If I was going to play in college someday, this is the position I would play.

Our Championship Season

As I got ready for my junior season, we set our expectations very high. We had a lot of knowledge about the other top teams in the area. We knew what Vianney had, what Aquinas had, what Rosary had. We knew we would be in the mix at the end of the year. We were loaded. We had a strong bench, too.

We did a lot of scouting. We would go up north to Koch Park and watch Rosary, Aquinas and some of the Hazelwood schools play. We were wearing our Oakville letter jackets, you know with the "O" on it, and people would ask us "what's that zero on your jacket?" We would jokingly say, "You'll know. You'll know by the end of the season." We weren't cocky. We were just confident.

We only lost three games that year. We lost to St. Mary's at Carondelet Park (*we actually played them a week later and beat them, but they were a very good team*). Our other losses were in penalty kicks, one against Bayless and the other against Vianney.

Defensively, we were very strong. We allowed just 11 goals in 28 games and I had 17 shutouts. I had a good season, but I have to credit my backs for our success. I had a special connection with our defenders — Kurt Billmeyer, Bill Colletta, Dominic Barczewski and Roger Schallom — and Gary Ullo controlled the midfield. It was just a unique trust that we had in each other. I would say we had the strongest defense in the state. Other teams had good goalies and decent defense, but ours was the best.

We won 23 games and tied two, which was by far the best record in the short history of our school at the time. One of our ties came against Roosevelt, a city school that was not even close to being one of the top teams in the area. I think it was a scoreless tie after regulation time and our coach — "Bokes" — wants to play overtime. We're looking around and the whole Roosevelt team is on the bus already. I think they wanted to see in the newspapers that they tied Oakville. Their coach told them we're going to play overtime, but the Roosevelt players were like, "Can't do it, coach. I've got to go to work." They came up with all kinds of excuses. It was an absolute riot.

Just before the state playoffs, Bokes brought two freshmen up to the varsity — Kenny Bromeier and Mike Dolan. They brought a lot of energy. Guys we brought off the bench would run their butts off. What we lacked in ability we made up for with hustle and hard work.

We had no easy path to the state final. We had to beat St. Mary's, DuBourg, Vianney and SLUH (*St. Louis U. High*). But we loved our spot. We were never No. 1 in the area rankings. We weren't one of the teams people tried to pick off.

After beating SLUH in the semifinal match, we knew we would be the underdog against Rosary in the state championship game. They had some great players like Don Ebert, Pat Howley and Terry Trushel. But we beat Rosary at the beginning of the year in the CYC Tournament. That gave us the boost we needed. We competed very well against good teams.

I remember practicing the day before the state final. It was a Friday afternoon and we were thinking, "wow, there's only two teams in the state practicing today…

and we're one of them." One of our players, Sean Hogan, made an "OSH #1" in the dirt. I think that cut some of the tension.

One thing I remember about the day of the state final was I wore another player's shoes. Mark Vonder Haar had a brand new pair of Puma King Pele soccer shoes. I told Mark I have to wear those shoes. I put those on and I felt 8 feet tall. They fit like a glove. That was the only game I ever wore Puma soccer shoes; I usually wore adidas. I was like, "wow, these are great." I also wore white adidas shorts, size 7, three red stripes, and then I wore a yellow shirt that I liked. It had a blue stripe down the side. I felt confident. I was ready to go.

On the day of the game the conditions were not great. It was a dirt field at O'Fallon Tech and the ball was bouncing all over the place. They had a lot of chances in the first half. I had to get over their heads on some crosses. I got off to a good start, a good rhythm. I could see that they were frustrated as we went into halftime with a 0-0 score. We knew we could win this thing. We were still competing.

I don't think we had a lot of direct shots, but we finally scored in the second half off a corner kick. Our freshmen forwards were running near post, there were guys running and bodies flying around in there. Finally, the ball went off Kenny Bromeier's knee into the goal and all I saw was our hands go up.

I knew they would be coming at us, and the pressure started coming constantly. I was able to get to some crosses, Bill Colletta cleared a ball off the line, I had to battle Don Ebert for some balls — and I came out on top. The scariest play came late in the game. I remember this shot I thought was going to beat me. The shot started to my right, but when I had full sight of it, it started bending back to my left. I'm like, "Oh sh__, that's behind me." I just lunged the other way. I got my hand on the ball and it just stuck to my hand right there on the goal line. Everyone talks about that save, but honest to God, it was luck.

So they're pouring on the pressure and we're just kicking balls out. As time was running down, the ball was at the other end of the field and Kurt Billmeyer turns around and whispers to me, "Jimmy, there's two minutes left." We were getting pretty excited, just hanging on.

The final whistle went off and all hell broke loose. We just beat Rosary 1-0 and won the state championship! Once we got the trophy, we took a lap around the field, acknowledging the fans. That was great. It's why you play. You want to win championships.

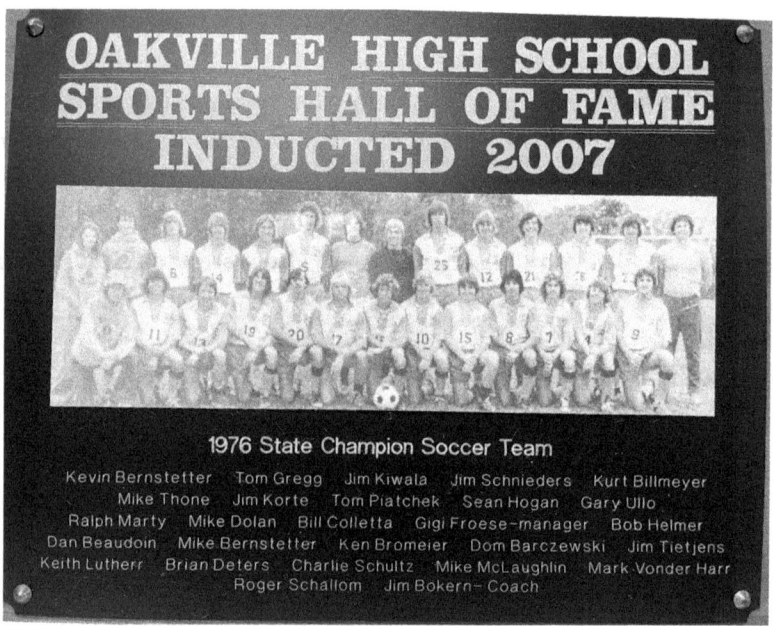

The 1976 state champions

I made 17 saves in that final game. I got a lot of credit for Oakville winning the state championship, which I think is complete BS. There were other players on our team that led the way. With myself, Gary, Dom, Kurt, Bill, we really had at least four players who were as good if not better than any other players in the state. I made all-state, Gary made all-state, Dominic made all-state, Kurt was honorable mention all-state, and Bill Colletta should have made all-state. None of us were fancy. We just did our job day in and day out.

An Assist to Coach Bokern

A lot of credit for our success goes to our coach, Jim Bokern. We all knew he played for the St. Louis Stars of the North American Soccer League. Just the fact that he was a professional soccer player who won three national championships as a player at St. Louis University gave him instant credibility with us. We bought into everything he said — hook, line and sinker.

Bokes, who was only about 24 when I joined varsity as a sophomore, liked to have fun. But he trained us very hard. He wanted us to be the fittest team in the state, and we were. Everything we did at practice was competitive. He wanted you to win, whether it was sprints, shuttles, short shuttles, long shuttles. You could feel the energy in the line. It rubbed off on everyone.

You had the non-starters working just as hard as the starters. Everyone pushed each other, a lot of physical training, a lot of soccer-related training. Back then you didn't see a lot of that. Bokes brought that from the Stars. Some of the coaches he had were international coaches, so he brought a lot of that into our program. We were in great shape. No one would outwork us in a game.

We practiced over at Bernard (*now a middle school in the Mehlville School District*). Bokes had this obstacle course we used to run through that was slightly over a mile. It went through the woods that were there before the new houses were built. He would have us do that at the beginning or sometimes the end of practice. And it was tough — I mean, it was an all-out sprint for some of us. I would look at the last quarter mile and give it everything I could.

We would also go down to Francis Field (*at Washington University*) and watch Bokes play for the Stars. It was a cool feeling being a high school player and having your coach down there playing for a professional team. After the games, we would wait for him outside the locker room and he would introduce us to some of the other players. I would always be looking for the goalies. He introduced me once to Lenny "James" Bond, the Stars goalkeeper. He would say, "Hey Tietj, I want you to meet our goalie." That's the equivalent of the Cardinals manager saying, "hey, come over here, I want you to meet Lou Brock. Hey Lou, this is my left fielder."

The Stars had good players from St. Louis at that time — Al Trost, Gary Rensing, Denny Vaninger, Larry Hausmann. Just to be able to get close to those guys was pretty cool.

Bokes also did things to build our confidence. I didn't enjoy talking to the newspaper reporters in those days. But whenever I was within earshot of Bokern being interviewed, he always made sure to say something positive about me. The day we won state, he told a reporter that I was the best high school goalkeeper he had ever seen. "I've never seen a kid with such poise," he said. "He could be playing for any number of college teams right now."

I think he was doing that to build up my confidence. Off the field, I was shy. But he believed in me. That just motivated me. I went from second tier to top tier among goalkeepers. That was because of his belief and his confidence in me. My willingness to accept that just challenged me to work that much harder.

Jim was a newlywed at that time, too. We would go over to their house on the weekends and play cards, have snacks. There were other times we would go over for a barbecue. That just speaks to the friendship and mutual respect we had for each other.

That was a special group of guys. Many of us went on to play in college. Some of us even played professionally. But if you ask each one of us what was our most satisfying soccer experience, the answer would be the same — winning the 1976 state championship.

Chapter 3

International Soccer

Right after we won the state championship my junior year, I was invited by Rick Benben, the assistant coach at SIU-Edwardsville, to go on a trip to Scotland with a bunch of players from the north side — Aquinas, Rosary, a couple of Hazelwood guys. He was taking a group of teams in three different age groups and he asked me to be their goalkeeper.

Our team was the "St. Louis Wanderers." Not only were we representing St. Louis, but we were the only team there from the United States. We played in Cowal, Scotland in a tournament called the Cowal International Youth Soccer Festival. It was a prestigious tournament. It was beyond me how this tournament on this tiny island off the coast of Scotland could be big. But it was.

We were taking the tournament by storm. We were breezing through and then we played Cowal in the final match. We controlled the game; we just couldn't score. They got a penalty kick on a questionable call late in the game and we lost, 1-0. I was so upset that I got a red card after the game was over. That was the only red card I ever got in my life.

After the game, they had a ceremony and handed out trophies. I thought I had a good tournament, but I didn't think they would give an award to a goalie. But they said, "winner of the award for most promising player, from the St. Louie Wanderers, Jimmy Tietjens."

It was an honor to receive this beautiful silver trophy. There were a couple of English magazines that mentioned that I had a good tournament. They wrote articles that said things like, "one player that impressed at the tournament was

Jimmy Tietjens from the St. Louie Wanderers. He managed his penalty area very well, was quick, confident, strong hands…"

That was my first experience playing soccer out of the country. It was a great time.

National Team Comes Calling

It was after we got back from Scotland when calls started coming in from the U.S. Soccer Federation. St. Louis had a lot of credibility on the national level, and coaches on the national team would get recommendations on players. My name was on a list of players being considered for the national team. I'm sure making all-state and then going on the trip to Scotland helped a lot.

I remember coming home from school and my mom told me a coach called from the U.S. Federation and he wants me to call him back. I couldn't get on the phone fast enough. I was being asked to try out for the youth national team.

We had different coaches over time. The highest coach was Walt Chyzowych, the director of coaching for the U.S. Federation. Walt was energetic, players loved him, demanded respect, just an easy guy to play for. Another top coach was Bob Gansler. He was a great player in his day, a wonderful coach who knew the game well. They were the senior national team coaches.

I spoke to Walt on the phone. I spoke to Bob Gansler on the phone. I also talked to Bill Muse, who worked at Princeton and coached the U.S. youth team. You're never automatically on the team, they're just inviting you to camp. They would bring in different players to see who might be able to help the national team, and always at least two goalkeepers. I always tried to approach it as if the job was mine. I was never given the job. I just felt, at that point, I earned the job.

So, I was selected for the U.S. Under-17 national team in early 1977. I wasn't the only player from St. Louis to get selected. We had myself, Perry Van Der Beck and John Hayes — all of us from St. Louis — all on the national team. Every time we would travel, we would get together about two weeks ahead of time and train.

One of our first tournaments was in Monte Carlo. That was an incredible tournament. We played France, Spain, Germany and Russia. We lost all four games, but we competed really hard in each of those games. Three games were close; we lost each one by a goal. The fourth game — we played Russia — they blew us out. It was 0-0 at halftime and we thought, "we're in this game, we could win this." They came out in the second half and they were buzzing all over the place, blasting balls at me. I think the final score was like 3 or 4 to nothing. They just took it to us.

That summer of '77 was an exciting time for me because it was the first time I got to travel abroad and really see Europe. We went to Holland, Italy, Switzerland, France, Germany. We were training in '77 to qualify for the Youth World Cup. We would go to big cities in Germany and play local all-star teams. I don't remember us losing any of those games. We didn't allow many goals.

I was very confident on the international level. We were playing against players the same age as us, and I don't remember anytime we were playing another country that I felt I wasn't better than that team's goalie. I thought at one point — at this age level — I may be the best in the world. That's a tall thought, but I had that kind of confidence. I wasn't intimidated. Neither was anyone else on our team.

Johnny Hayes, who was my roommate (*and a future All-American at St. Louis University*), was an amazing forward. He wasn't intimidated. That was our approach, our mindset. But there's a funny story about Johnny. Bill Muse, our head coach, was somebody I respected tremendously. We would train at his school before heading out for a tournament. It was about a two-hour drive to Kennedy Airport, where we would get on a plane and go to another country.

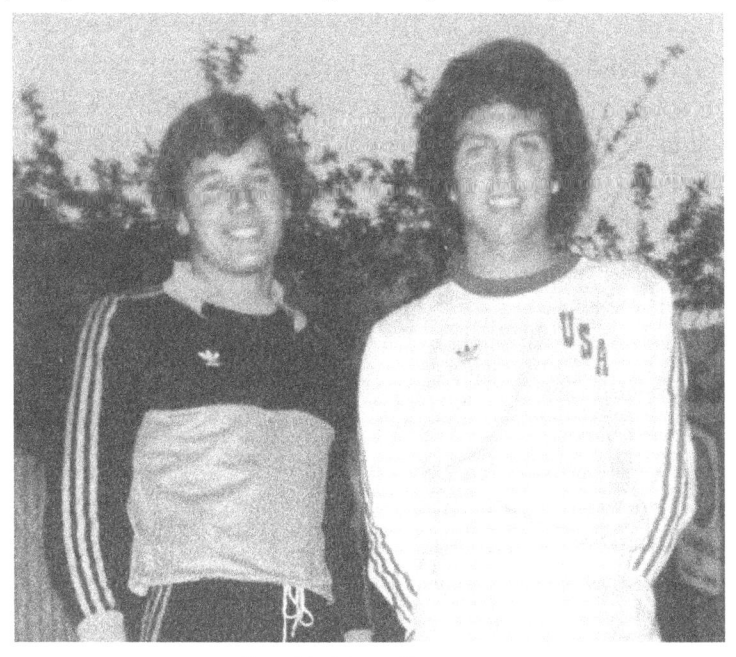

Jim with Johnny Hayes

I remember one trip we were going on, we stopped at a rest stop to use the restroom and then everyone got back on the bus. You were supposed to be in charge of your roommate — Johnny was mine — well, the bus took off and Johnny wasn't on it. We were an hour out when we discovered Johnny was not on the bus. "Where's Hayzer?" It then became a joke. Johnny was always picking his hair; he had this sort of long frizzy hair. Someone said, "he's still in the bathroom shaping his hair."

The coaches were not happy. We stopped in front of a bar in a little town, a little tavern. The coach went in and got a hold of somebody and they drove Johnny out to meet us. Think about how hard that was. Can you imagine Johnny at the rest stop? He comes out and the bus is gone? Johnny's 17, probably never been out of St. Louis, so that was kind of exciting. We were kids. We just laughed.

There was another time in Germany when we had just got in on a long flight from Kennedy and we had jet lag. We were just worn out. We were supposed to train at this field that was probably more than two miles away. Well, the goalies were roomed together — Barry Stringfeld was the other goalie — and we had the balls, two big ball bags. We fell asleep and then finally woke up after the team had left for practice. "Barry, holy crap, we're late," I said. "And they don't have any balls."

We had to ask people if they knew where the team went (*of course, we don't speak German*). So, this is not good, we gotta run, and it's at least two miles to the field. We're lugging these big ball bags. It's the longest I ran at one time. "Barry, we gotta step it up," I said. "Coach is not going to be happy." We finally got there and I think they got some balls from the club where they were practicing. The guys were giving us a hard time, but the coaches were smart. They figured we already ran a couple of miles. They appreciated that we got ourselves there on our own. It was sink or swim. You're not at home. Your parents aren't there to take care of you. It was a growing experience.

I remember another time playing in Switzerland. We were playing in a stadium that was used in the 1954 World Cup. The fans always got into the American teams — in a good way. They were right down near the field. Someone behind the goal brought some dollar bills to the game and he was putting them on the goal line. He would say, "Hey, pay you some money if you let a goal in." They weren't scoring and I was playing well. I went back there, picked up the money and put it in my shorts. I just said, "hey, thank you." We were having fun. The fans were having fun. It was just a fun atmosphere, so easy to play in.

After the game, you would have dinner with the other team. They were excited to host you. We would see these guys on their national teams and we would get to know these guys. It was just an incredible experience for a 17-year old. I think back about what I learned about the people, the cultures, and how much I loved meeting people.

A Tough Decision

After that exciting summer, my intention was to play my senior year at Oakville. But I hurt my ankle at the beginning of the season. I remember playing in a game against CBC and not being able to move. The national team had a qualifying tournament coming up later that year, and I wanted to be ready for that, so I made the decision to shut it down and stop playing for Oakville.

I told Jim Bokern, and obviously he was not happy. I had a lot of success with the national team, and I was their No. 1 goalkeeper. Winning the state championship at Oakville with the guys I was with the year before were the guys I was close to. I felt like that team had moved on and I needed to be true to the national team. I would have loved to play my whole senior year at Oakville, but I felt an obligation to the national team because we were getting ready for Youth World Cup qualifying.

I understood that my decision wasn't fair to my teammates here (*at Oakville*). But, at that point, my mission was to try to become a better goalie. I knew with the national team I had the best chance of doing that.

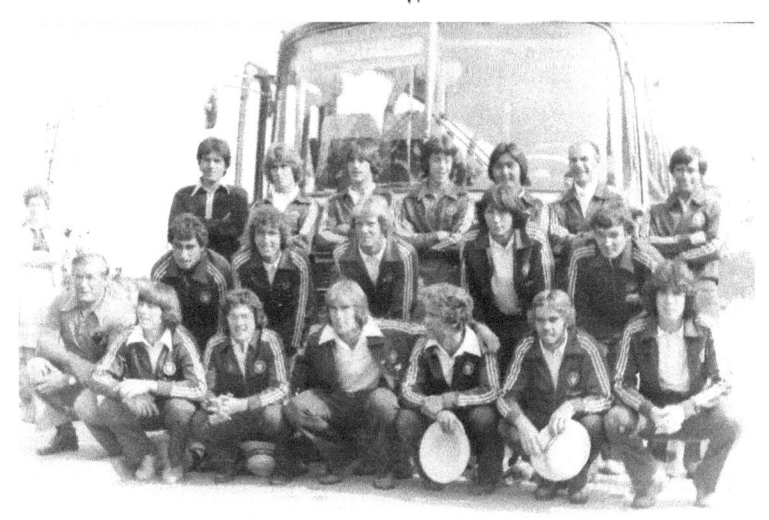

U.S. youth national team

Youth World Cup Qualifiers

The qualifying games for the Youth World Cup were in Honduras. We played Honduras, Canada, Costa Rica, and Trinidad and Tobago. We stayed in the hills at a nun's convent, and we had guards with us. We would go to practices or games in a school bus and there would be a guy in fatigues in the front of the bus and a guy in fatigues in the back of the bus… with machine guns, so it was kind of eye-opening for a 17-year old kid.

We won our first two games against Costa Rica and Trinidad and Tobago, we tied Canada, and then we played Honduras. We played in a stadium that seated 50,000 people and it was full when we played Honduras. We needed to win that game to advance to the next group. We had them tied 0-0. We played 90 minutes and they were all over us. They were pouring it on, and it was just a matter of time before they scored.

The referee just kept letting the game go on and on. Our coaches are looking at their watches. We're in the 58th minute of the second half and the half is supposed to be 45 minutes. The coaches were like, "What's going on here?" Well, they scored in the 58th minute of the half. As soon as we centered off, the ref blew the whistle and the game was over. Our coach told us the second half was 58 minutes. I just know it felt like forever.

Earlier that week we went to a party. They had some girls from Honduras there and they were telling us that there were three guys on the Honduran team that were 21. They were saying, "the captain, he's like a man, he's 21." But that's how it was over there. They had fake passports. You played by their rules. Overall, it was a successful trip, but we got our eyes opened to what can happen to you when you play in Central America.

We continued to play some youth tournaments. There were a lot of trips. I think my senior year I missed about 50 days of school. The school was really good about it. They worked with me. I did take books with me on the trips, not that I opened them a great deal. But the teachers were very good about it. I missed my graduation, but they helped me with my credits.

The Olympic Pool

At this point, it became the 1980 Olympic team. We had a pool of 35 to 40 players, maybe four or five goalies. I was not picked to be part of the final 20 for the Olympic team. I had my chance. I had my ups and downs. I just didn't adjust as well as I should have. Dave Brcic, from St. Louis, was on the Olympic team and he was a strong goalie. I was with him on multiple trips, always as the backup. Then there was Paul Coffee from Santa Clara. In those days, Paul was playing professionally. Dave was, too. I went on a lot of trips with those guys but never earned a spot.

One year after we won a tournament in Switzerland, the coaches took us to Puerto Rico for a series of games. To be honest, it was kind of a vacation. The coaches brought their wives, and we played just two games in Puerto Rico. We traveled to this one game in a small town. We traveled on a school bus to this old city with one way streets. We got to the field and we started playing the game.

Dave Brcic was in goal. We're scoring goals left and right, and every time we score a goal, the referee is saying it's offside. I think we scored four or five goals quickly in the first half that were called back. Players were getting frustrated, the coaches were getting frustrated. Don Ebert (*another player from St. Louis*) is in a tussle with someone from the other team. This was supposed to be a Friendly, but there's a scuffle on the field. Next thing you know there's people coming out of the stands. I look behind me and I see men charging towards the field. The coach is screaming, "Get on the bus."

We start running for the bus. Fortunately, the coaches' wives never got off the bus. We get on the bus and they're throwing rocks at us. One rock hit the window and it sounded like a gun pop. That's when I got down on the floor and away from the windows. The bus driver, he's just tearing through the crowd. He makes a left turn down a one-way street. We're going the opposite way to get back. We're like, "what the hell is he doing?"

We have to turn around and go back through this crowd. He turns around and we go right past the stadium. We're down and keeping our mouths shut. He's going as fast as he can. Fortunately, we got back to the hotel in one piece.

I had some scary moments playing internationally, but I wouldn't trade that experience for anything.

Chapter 4

Choosing St. Louis U.

The North American Soccer League held the first-ever draft of high school players in January of 1978. Perry Van Der Beck of Aquinas went No. 1 to the Tampa Bay Rowdies. I went No. 2 to the California Surf. For me, it was kind of an honor to be picked No. 2 in the first high school draft. I mean, wow, I'm still 17, just a kid, thinking it's a pretty cool deal.

The Surf also drafted Johnny Hayes, who was from Aquinas. Myself and Johnny were roommates on the U.S. national team, so we knew each other very well. They told us they would fly us out there to train and visit with the team. We stayed in a Best Western right near Disneyland. We were only there for about two and a

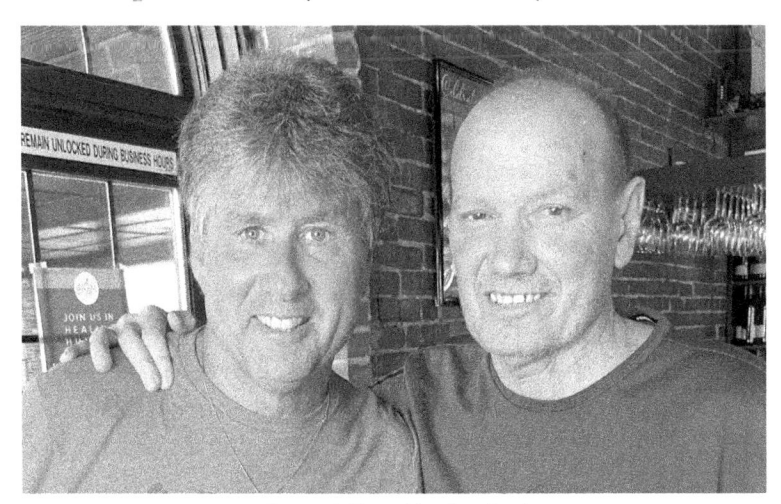

Jim with Perry Van Der Beck

half days. We trained one day in a park, about 12 to 14 guys playing small-sided games with small goals. We had a second training session that was indoors, but both training sessions went well for Johnny and myself.

Johnny was a cut above everyone else. He was a pure goal scorer. If he had the right people feeding him the ball, he could put it in the back of the net. Johnny was incredibly quick and incredibly fast with the ball.

We both thought we could do this, but for me it was just too big of a step. Neither of us had any intention of going pro at that time. We had both already committed to St. Louis U. I remember calling the general manager and thanking him for bringing me out and showing me around. I thought at that point in time it was best for me to go to college.

Becoming A Billiken

I started getting recruited my junior year. I had all kinds of offers from outside the state, but I never really considered them seriously. I had my sights set on SLU. When I was watching college soccer in St. Louis, that was the place to go.

I remember when I committed to SLU. Jim Bokern, who played on three national championship teams at SLU, was so proud that I decided to go there. He gave me this light blue jacket that he had from his playing days at SLU. It had the Billiken logo on it. It was a pretty cool thing.

When I was being recruited, Harry Keough, SLU's head coach, would come out to my house with his assistants, Miguel de Lima and Val Pelizzaro. Miguel was Harry's longtime friend from Brazil who was also a goalkeeper. Everyone knew Miguel. He was a first-team player in the Brazilian national program. He had all kinds of goalkeeping knowledge. My belief was he was going to be my goalkeeping coach at SLU.

There were times that summer before my freshman year I would meet Miguel at Forest Park and train there. We did a lot of fitness training, a lot of leg and foot-speed drills. If you have good hands, you can be a good goalkeeper, but it's really from the waist down. It's your leg strength. It's your foot quickness that gets you to balls.

It was a thrill to work out with him. I remember we would run sprints from the goal line to midfield, and then we would do the full length of the field. We would sprint and then jog back. We would do 12 sets of that. I mean, that's a lot of running. He just pushed you. You knew that he was successful in Brazil, so he had instant credibility. You wanted to do whatever he asked you to do.

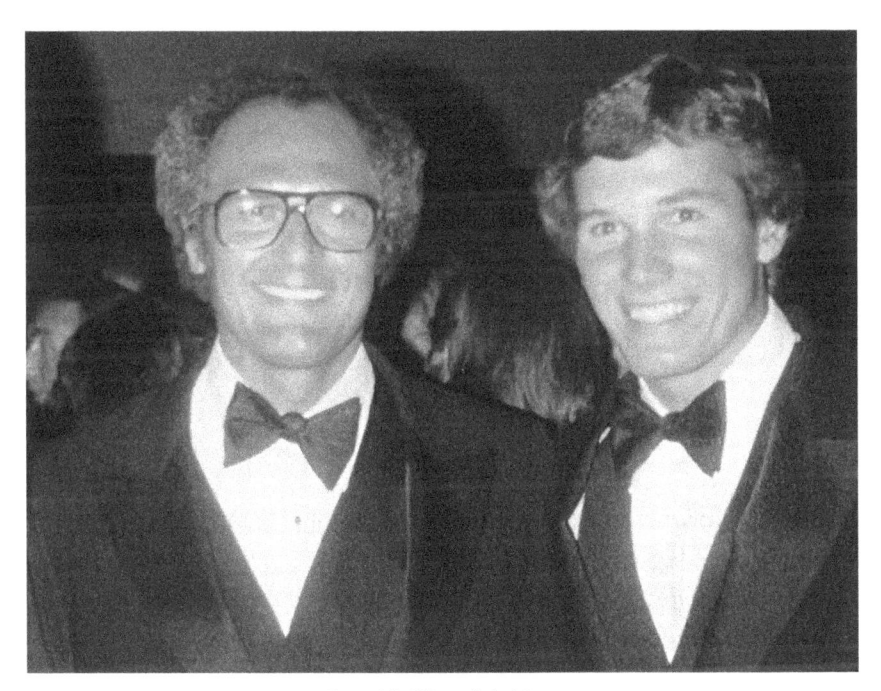

Jim with Miguel de Lima

Playing with the national team and then working out with Miguel, I grew as a player. I was polishing my skills. I was never a flashy goalie. I was someone who used my foot speed, my reflexes, I had good hands. I could be in the right position to make the game look easy. And that comes from training.

What happened — and it was kind of a big deal for me — was Miguel was offered a job with the New York Cosmos. That's how much he was respected in the U.S. He took the job and no longer was in the mix at SLU, so that was a disappointment to me.

A New Goalkeeping Coach

Harry went on to hire a guy by the name of Skip Grossman as the new goalkeeping coach. Skip was good friends with Miguel. He was a good goalkeeping coach. He wasn't Miguel, but he was good. My relationship with Skip was OK. It wasn't as strong as it would have been with Miguel, but it wasn't bad.

I trained hard and was excited to play for SLU. I had a good freshman year. I had 107 saves, which I think still ranks among the top five single-season totals among SLU goalies. We played good teams and I built up some respect. I really enjoyed playing with those players, the Ty Keoughs and Larry Hulcers of the world. I had

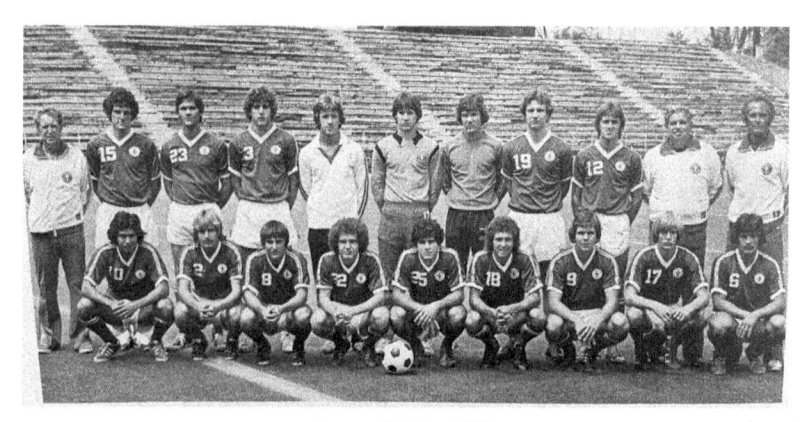

Jim at SLU in 1978

a lot of respect for them, both players on the national team, both on the Olympic team. They played big-time international games.

I don't know why, but I didn't go into my sophomore year with the same excitement that I had going into my freshman year. Maybe it's because we lost some players from my freshman year, but I didn't feel the environment was one in which I could excel. I made some mistakes, but I played well enough in some games to be nominated for All-American honors (*I made second team*). I was kind of surprised I got it, although I did finish the season with 118 saves.

However, I didn't feel a lot of growth as a goalkeeper. I certainly wasn't performing to expectations. I was very disappointed in myself. For the first time ever in my years of playing soccer, I lost some confidence. It seemed as the year went on, it got worse.

The Final Straw

In the final game of the year, I was benched. It was myself and the other goalie, Dale Smith, who was a very good goalie from one of the Parkway schools (*Parkway West*). Skip told us the position for the final game was still to be determined. He said, "We're going to watch training this week and see how you train, and that's how it will be determined."

That was kind of a shock to me. I wasn't happy. I also knew I wanted to train my ass off and prove that I should be the choice. I'm sure Dale felt the same way. So I had a good week of training and felt I earned the position, but I was told I was not going to play. Dale would be playing. I was not happy, but I kept my mouth shut. I tried to be a team player.

Dale was a class guy. Even when they told me I wasn't going to be playing, when the conversation was over I turned around and walked to my car. Dale ran up to me before I could leave and told me he was sorry. I said, "Dale, that's fine. I'll be behind you." I wanted the team to win.

So we're playing SIU-Edwardsville in the national playoffs. Dale played well, but SIU won on a penalty kick. I tried to tell Dale what side (*Don*) Ebert would go to, and he went to that side. Dale almost got it, but he didn't.

Certainly, I wanted the team to go on. But some things didn't sit well with me in how that whole situation was handled. I still wanted to play professionally, and I felt if I stayed there any longer, I could continue to go downhill.

After that game, I stayed in the locker room until everyone was gone. I talked to Harry by myself and let him know I didn't like the way things were handled. It wasn't a heated conversation. I just wanted to let him know how I felt. At the end of the day, he's the coach. He made some statements to me that he thought I wasn't on my game. He thought the team needed a change. I accepted it, but I pretty much decided at that point that was it for me at SLU.

A month or so later, I went to the athletic director and told him I was leaving SLU and planned to turn pro. I did not tell Harry that I was leaving. As I look back on it, I wish I would have told Harry personally. Harry deserved that respect — he earned it. As I got older, I just really wish I would have handled it in a different way.

Chapter 5

Playing Pro Soccer

Once I left SLU, I made myself available for the NASL supplemental draft. It was a bigger deal than I thought because you can't go back to college once you declare for the draft. If you don't get picked, you're out.

Fortunately, I was picked by the Fort Lauderdale Strikers. It was kind of a surprise because I didn't know if there was anyone down there that knew me. Apparently, someone did. I had to go down there and compete hard for my job. They already had two goalies. The starter was Arnie Mausser, who was one of the

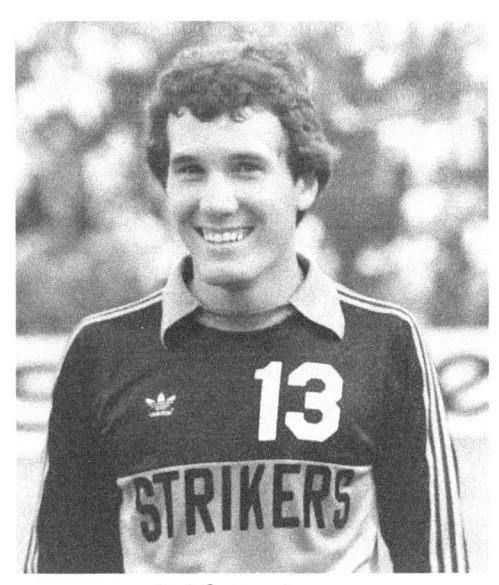

Jim's first pro team

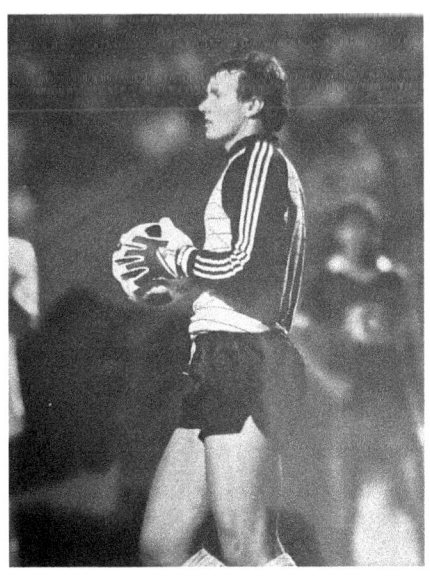

Jim with Fort Lauderdale

two U.S. national team goalies. He was there with another player who came from Baltimore, Steve Zerhusen. He had been on the team, but at that time, Steve had back surgery and he was out for most of the season.

So, it was myself and another young kid from Canada. I was competing with the Canadian kid for the back-up position, and I knew right away that I could win out over him. Eventually, I ended up making the team. It was myself and Arnie as the team's goalkeepers.

We had a coach from Holland, Cor van der hart. He liked how I played and how I practiced. He liked my work ethic. I showed the skills and confidence in practice. He could see that I could play.

However, Cor had his heart set on bringing in an experienced goalkeeper from Holland, Jan van Beveren. Jan played for an Einhoven team that won the Dutch first division championship several times. He came over here and he was the real deal. I had never seen a goalie who had the range to get out, start diving, and get to balls. It came from his quick feet. He had amazing power in his legs. Beyond that, his reflexes were amazing.

Arnie moved on to another team, so Jan started most of the games. I hardly played. My first game was against Chicago at the old Comiskey Stadium. We lost that one, 3-1. Three days later, I played in a victory at home against Portland. Those were the only two games I played that year.

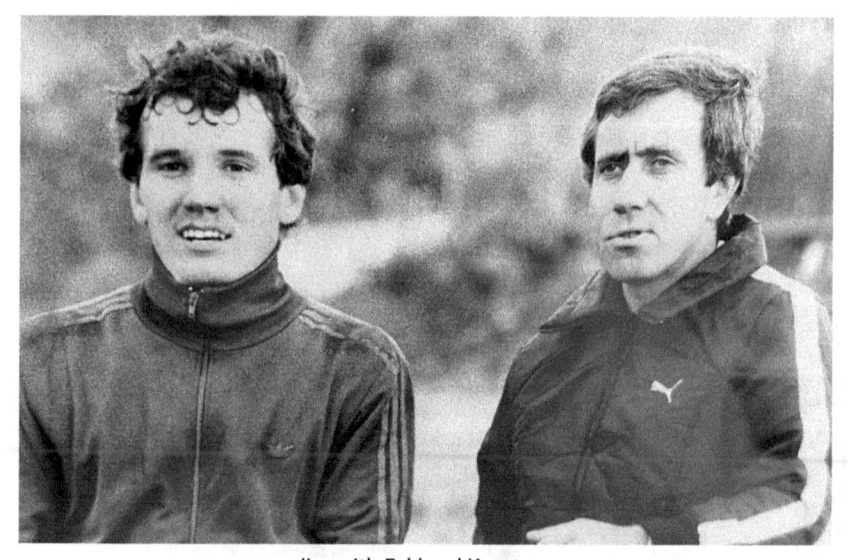

Jim with Eckhard Krautzun

Our team went to Soccer Bowl '80 that year. We played the New York Cosmos in Washington, DC in front of more than 50,000 people at RFK Stadium. Jim McKay was covering the game for ABC. He came up to me in the locker room before the game and introduced himself. He even knew my name, so obviously he studied up on the players.

The Cosmos didn't have Pele then, but they did have (Franz) Beckenbauer and (Giorgio) Chinaglia. We were never really in the game. The Cosmos won, 3-0.

A Coaching Change

That spring, our Dutch coach got fired and they brought in a German coach by the name of Eckhard Krautzun. Right away, I could tell Eckhard respected me a lot. He saw that I had potential. They were confident that if something happened to Jan, they have a guy who knows what he's doing. But I think Jan wound up playing every game that year.

We had several German players on the team, the most popular being Gerd Muller. Everyone who played soccer in my era knows who Gerd Muller is. He is one of the greatest goal scorers in the history of the sport; he scored 14 goals in two World Cups. When he passed away in 2021, the country was in mourning for a week.

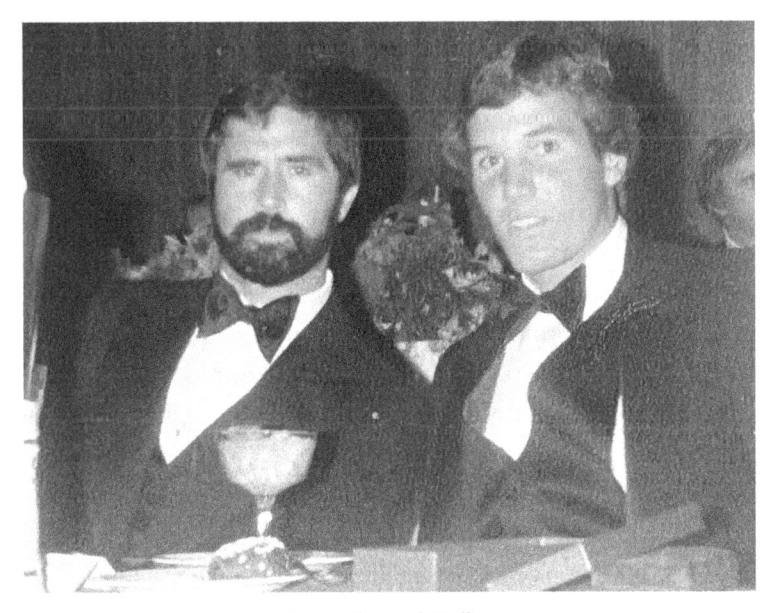

Jim with Gerd Muller

I remember my first training session after I got drafted. Gerd Muller was there and I was wearing his brand of shoes — Gerd Muller Golds. I'm 20 years old and this is a guy I watched on TV when I was 10. He was a legend. Once I was on the team with him, though, I wasn't intimidated. We played a short-sided game (*about eight players on a side*) and Gerd played sweeper in front of me. I remember making one very good save. Gerd's like, "Schon, Jimmy, Schon. Good. Good." He was always nice to me. He just felt comfortable with the American kids.

We had other great players. Ray Hudson, an Englishman who played for Newcastle United, was a really talented midfielder. Ray was always able to thread the needle to Gerd. If you get the ball to Gerd in the 18-yard box, he's generally going to put it away. And then we had another player named Teofilo Cubillas from Peru. His nickname was El Nene (*The Kid*). At one time some were comparing Nene to Pele, just an amazing player with so much skill and ability.

A Trip to Germany

Jan played pretty much every game the next three seasons, but there were still some memorable moments for me. We did a postseason tour of Germany with the Strikers after the '81 season. We played four or five games — I'd play a half, Jan would play a half — I'm pretty sure we never lost. The German Bundesliga was in season, so we were just playing all-star teams from different areas in Germany.

We were going to watch a game in Borussia Monchengladbach. They were a big-time team in the Bundesliga, them and Bayern Munich. We were taking our team bus to the game. When we got to the stadium, the game had already started. Our German coach wants to park our bus inside the stadium on the football grounds, where the away team usually parks the bus. Our coach gets off the bus and talks to the gatekeeper, and the gatekeeper is not having any of it whatsoever.

Now we're laughing because he's telling us how well known he is in Germany. He gets on the bus and is kind of embarrassed. Thomas Rongen, one of our Dutch players, is like, "Coach, is everything OK? Is there anything I can do, coach?" "No, Thomas. I have it under control." But really, he's in the shits because they're not letting him into the game.

So Gerd stands up. Remember, Gerd is a legend in Germany, right? He turns around, kinda shy, looks at us, "Guys, guys, should I?" We're all saying, "Gerd, Gerd, do something." "Nah, I don't want to embarrass him… Aw, OK."

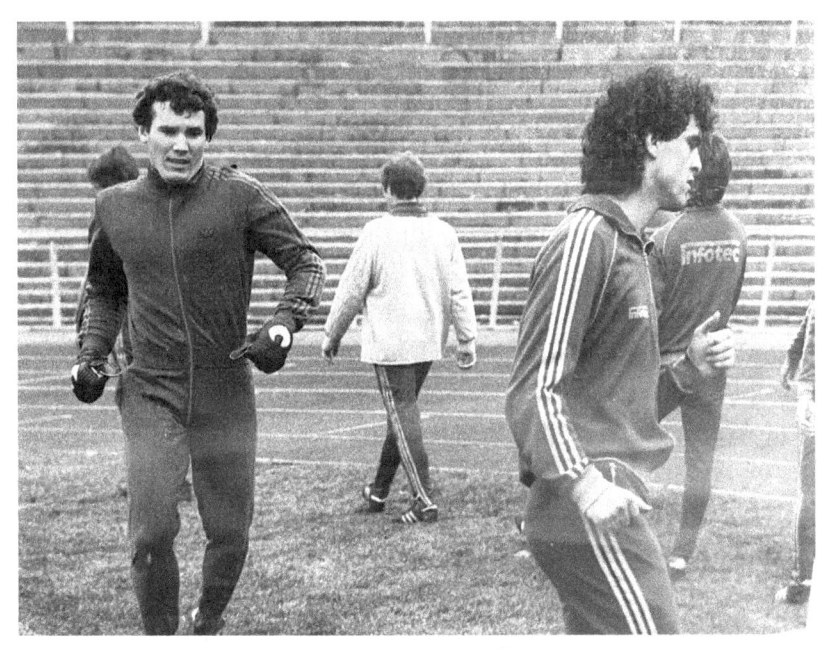

Jim training with Eintracht Frankfurt in Germany

So Gerd gets off the bus, walks over to the gatekeeper. The gatekeeper — his eyes are as big as oranges — just opens the gate and in comes the bus. But it gets better. Our seats were across the field, so we had to walk past the goal, halfway up the field before we could get to our seats. The fans are starting to make some noise because they see Gerd on the field. Even some of the players on the field are turning around to see what's going on.

The crowd is now chanting his name, "Mul-ler, Mul-ler"... I'm on Gerd's left, Bobby Meschbach, who played at Indiana, is on his right. The ball goes out of bounds and play stops for 30, 40 seconds. We've got our hands on Gerd's shoulders and we're waving to the crowd. I'm only 21, and this is just unbelievable. It's something I'll never forget.

Training in Germany

The best experience I had, though, was in the fall of '82. We had another German player on the team, Bernd Holzenbein. Bernd was another legend; he played on the '74 German team with Gerd that won the World Cup. Bernd and I became friends, so one day I told him that I really want to go to Germany in the offseason and stay there for a few months and train. He said, "Jimmy, I can arrange that."

So he arranged it. I went over to train with his former team, Eintracht Frankfurt. Bernd, who was a legend in Frankfurt, introduced me to everyone on the team. He said, "this is my friend Jimmy, he plays in America, he's very good…" They treated me like gold.

I stayed there for five weeks. I was — and I don't say this much — I was amazing. I could not believe it. I was playing with the first team and training with them. Everything just clicked. They're sending Bernd messages, "you know, this guy is unbelievable." There was no shyness about me. It was an unbelievable atmosphere. You just get into it, and I felt like one of them.

Newspapers in Germany were doing articles on me. One headline said "Florida Boy in Frankfurt" and had a picture of big oranges by me. They interviewed some of the other players and they were saying good things about me. Our Fort Lauderdale coach came to see me train one day. "Jimmy, they're telling me unbelievable things about you." I'm like, "I'm just doing what I do." That made me feel pretty good. These were experiences that just helped my game tremendously.

If I had to do it all over again, I would have probably tried to go to Germany, stayed there and played. I was young. I didn't think about that. I enjoyed living in Fort Lauderdale. You know, the beach. But if I had to do it over, that's what I would do. I would set my sights on Germany.

Trouble Indoors

The NASL had an indoor season for a couple years, so when I got back from Germany, I remember playing in an indoor game in Montreal. One reason I remember that game was because it was played in the Montreal Forum. They had all the Canadiens banners hanging from the rafters — Dryden, Cournoyer, Beliveau, Richard. It was unbelievable.

The game went to a shootout. This guy was dribbling in on me, he made a move around me. I made my move to get him, which I did. As soon as I went down, I just felt something pop in my leg. The trainer came out and I said, "I'm out." I knew right away.

It was a pretty serious injury, the anterior cruciate, a straight tear all the way through the ligament in my right knee. I went back to Fort Lauderdale and had surgery within a day or two. Our orthopedic surgeon was the Miami Dolphins surgeon, Dr. Dan Kanell (*his son Danny played quarterback at Florida State*). I became very close to him. He was an amazing doctor.

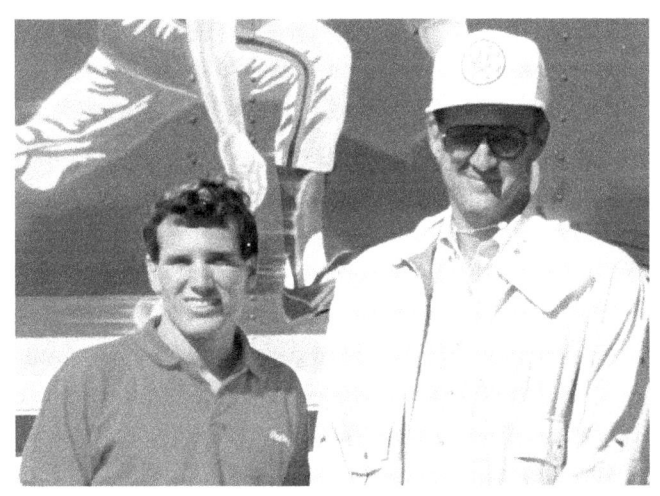

Jim with Dr. Kanell

So, here I am, 22 years old, and I'm rehabbing. A new coach came in from England, David Chadwick. This other goalie — Craig Scarpelli — and I would go at it. We competed hard with each other, and that's all good. Craig was a good guy, good goalie, competitive.

As we went into the spring of '83, they didn't need three goalies and they're trying to get rid of one of us. I remember when the coach called me and said they were going to let me go. Chadwick had coached Craig in the ASL (*American Soccer League*), so he kept Craig and put me on waivers.

I got picked up by the Kansas City Comets to play indoors, which I didn't really want to do. I played there for a year and I don't think I played more than five or six games. They had a smaller goalie by the name of Enzo DiPede, who was the No. 1 goalie. They didn't re-sign me the next season, so I went to try out for the Steamers in St. Louis. I played in a pre-season game against KC and we shut them out, but overall I didn't do very well. My leg was hurt. In the end, I didn't pass the physical, so I didn't make the team.

Opportunity in the USL

I went back down to Florida to see Dr. Kanell and get another surgery on my knee. The Strikers moved to Minnesota, but I heard Fort Lauderdale was starting this team down there in the USL (*United Soccer League*) called the Fort Lauderdale Sun. Keith Weller, who played for the Strikers, became the player-coach for the Sun and he asked me to be their goalkeeper. I saw Dr. Kanell in the fall of '83 and I knew I had time to rehab.

I know I had slowed down a little from my knee operations, but I did feel I was getting stronger. We had a really solid team in '84. We knew from the get-go that we had a pretty good chance of winning the league. I was the No. 1 goalie, we won the Southern Division and allowed just 34 goals in 24 games, the fewest in the league.

We beat Buffalo in the semifinal round of the playoffs and then it was us and Houston in the final. We lost on penalty kicks in the first game and beat them in the second game, so we had one more game to determine the champion.

I had a good game, their goalie had a good game. It ended in a 1-1 tie, so now we go to a shootout. It was 2-2 after five rounds and now nobody's scoring. I'm stopping theirs and he's stopping ours. I'm just thinking, "Something's gotta give. How long can I keep this up?" I still remember their ninth shooter hit a scorcher and, honestly, I barely got a finger on it. It didn't change the direction by more than two inches, but it was just enough. Finally, our ninth shooter scores and we win the shootout — and the league championship.

I was named the top goalkeeper of the playoffs and a first-team all-star goalie. It was a good feeling because I had been through a lot. To win a championship, it was just an amazing moment, to get the trophy and be able to hold it up there and jog around the field in front of our fans. I remember that night in the locker room. It had taken a long time to win a championship, and I just didn't want to leave. We were out all night and got to see the sun rise the next morning. It was a good time.

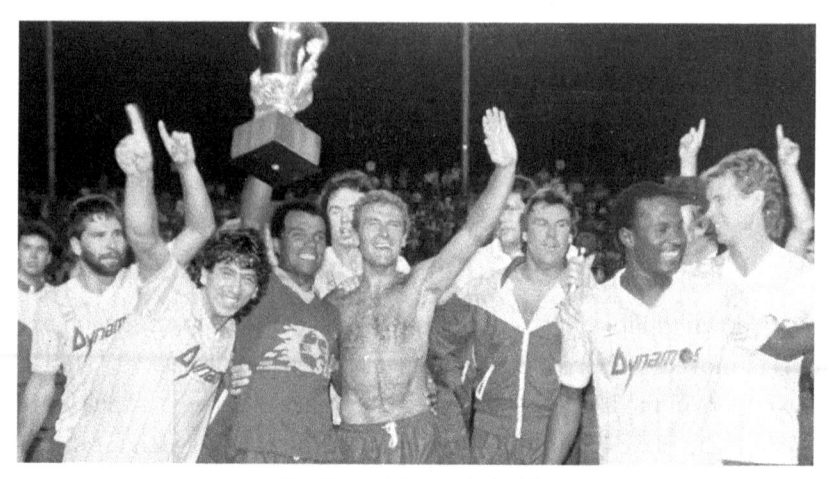

The Sun celebrate their title

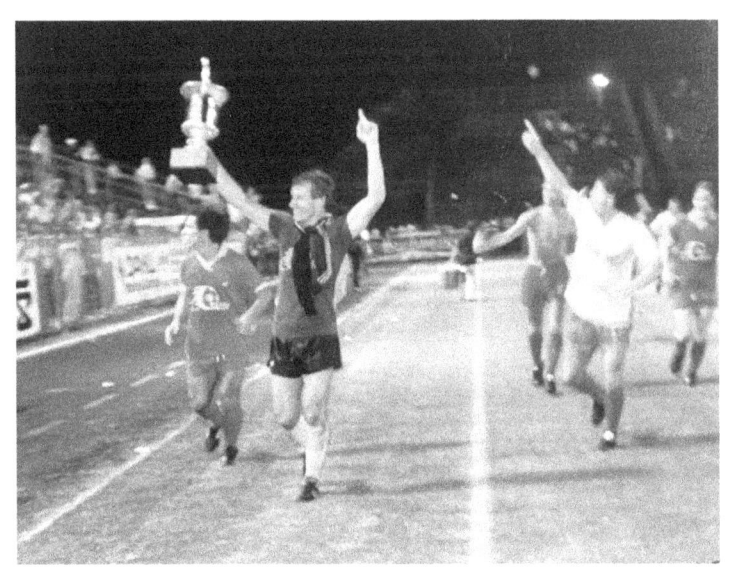

Jim hoists the trophy

We had a good team the next year. We picked up a great player from Holland, Johan Neeskens. Unfortunately, we got halfway through the season and the team folded. Our coach, Keith Weller, pulled a game together against the Haitian all-stars from Miami. They brought the gate receipts into the locker room after the game and we divided the money by player. I was one of the better known players, so I think I got $342.

That was a disappointing way to end my professional career, but I have to thank Keith Weller for giving me the chance to play and win a championship. It was a great experience.

Chapter 6

Caravan Man

After my last season in Fort Lauderdale, I had my third knee operation. I just felt, with three surgeries, maybe now is the time to finish school and get a real job. The NASL, for the most part, had folded. Some teams in the USL stayed in existence, but the one I was on in Fort Lauderdale didn't. It didn't look like I could continue to make a career out of soccer. I had my shot and did the best I could. I had some fun and that was it.

I came home to St. Louis and actually moved back in with my folks. I was still pretty young, about 25. A friend of mine's father owned a business called Fluid-Air Products. They sold spray paint equipment to the city and county and auto makers, all this equipment to paint streets, airplanes and cars. I was a manager of a small warehouse. It wasn't a high paying job, but I was able to pay my mom and step-dad a small amount of rent and have some money to go out on the weekends.

I knew I needed to go back to school and work towards my degree. I took some night courses while I was working at Fluid-Air and then I started going to Webster College (*now Webster University*). But then I found a really great opportunity. I was able to get what I considered to be a good job at Rawlings Sporting Goods. Mike Redohl's dad had a very good relationship with the human resources people at Rawlings, so he was able to talk to them and they brought me in for an interview.

I was fortunate that they had a job opening for a promotions manager on something called the Rawlings Sports Caravan. It was a big rig that pulled two connected trailers. One of the trailers was a Rawlings museum and the other was a workshop where you would make gloves and bats. I had to go to a truck driver training school for almost four months before I could get out on the road.

Every year we would tour the country and visit sporting goods dealers. We would go to every state and put on shows, like three or four hours, where people would come out and we would show them how we make gloves and bats. I was the glove master. If someone needed a glove re-strung, I knew how to do it. People would be in line for hours. At the end of the day, my fingers were tough from using leather all day.

Working With the Pros

We would also go to spring training and work with the pro ballplayers. We would spend about four weeks in Arizona and then drive to Florida to cover the teams there. The players that were under contract to Rawlings would generally start off the season with two gloves and break them in. Depending on the player, sometimes they might get three gloves. You got to know them a little bit personally.

When Ken Griffey Jr. was a rookie, I remember his first spring training. He rolled into camp in a white BMW with all the extras on it, like dark tinted windows and gold rims. He came out to the trailer one day and was very friendly. He had an old Rawlings 6-finger glove called the trapeze; it had a lot of lacing. He wanted me to

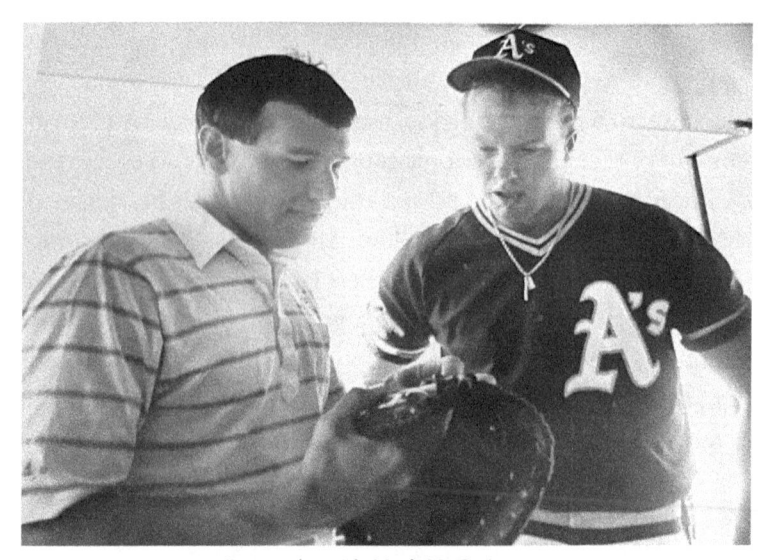

Jim works with Mark McGwire

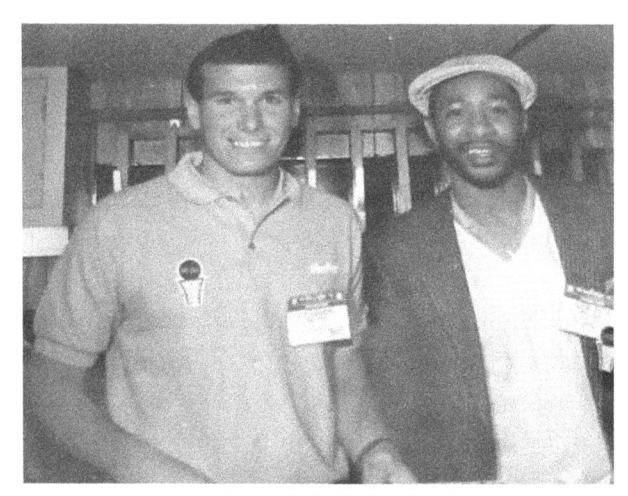

Jim with Ozzie Smith

re-lace his glove and put brown laces in a black glove. The way the lacing leather was tanned that year, it looked more like gold than it did brown. He liked the look of it.

So we started making those gloves with that blend of brown and gold lacing. A lot of different players caught on and started asking for the same thing, so I was putting a lot of brown/gold laces into black gloves. Mark McGwire came out to our truck one day. He had a black first baseman's mitt that had a panel that goes across the web ripped out. He asked if I could fix it. I told him I could, but I only have brown leather. So, I put the brown leather in it, I showed him the lacing, and he loved it. So, from then on, that's the way we would make it for him at our factory.

Ozzie Smith always liked a stiff glove. The way he played the game, Ozzie used his glove to guide the ball from his glove to his hand, not always catching it as much as guiding it in one movement. Just about every time I would see him he wanted me to re-do his glove. If you want a glove to be a little more stable, instead of getting a new glove, just put laces in it. When you put thick new laces in a glove, it's going to be stiff for probably six weeks.

I also got to know Tony Gwynn. Tony was a great guy, just a nice guy, always respectful to us. He always knew our names. But there was a line that I didn't cross. I never asked for autographs or anything like that.

Traveling Man

I was almost 27 when I started working at Rawlings, and it was a great job because I got to see a ton of the country. I'm talking from Los Angeles to San Francisco, up the Pacific Coast Highway to Oregon, make a right turn and go to Idaho, Montana, Wyoming, North Dakota, South Dakota. It was cool because these are places I normally would not get to see.

I remember doing a show in Wyoming. We were set up in a park and in the distance, probably a couple miles away, we saw two twin tornadoes. My first thought was, "wow, our truck is going to get destroyed." It took us about 10 minutes, if that, to shut everything down. There was a big maintenance building nearby in the park. They had a little basement, so we were able to go down there. Fortunately, the tornadoes never reached us. They got sucked right back up into the sky and just dissolved. That was scary.

The best part of the job, though, was just the opportunity to meet so many wonderful people. We got to know people so well we would go back to their stores the next year. So we had a lot of fun. It was a very cool experience.

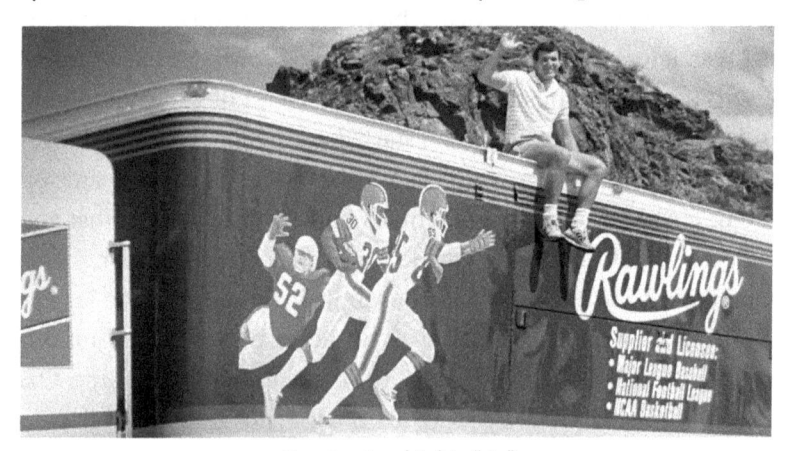

Jim sits atop his big "rig"

Chapter 7

Karen's Death

My sister Karen was first diagnosed with cardiomyopathy when I started working for Rawlings in the fall of 1986. I would go out to see her when she was a lieutenant in the Navy stationed in California. I would walk into buildings with her and I would see people jump up and salute her. I was so proud of her and what she had accomplished.

I remember right after graduating from truck driver training school — I had to drive the big rig for Rawlings — I flew out to San Francisco to see Karen. She had already been diagnosed and wasn't feeling well. One day we went over the Golden Gate Bridge to a spot where we climbed up a pretty big hill. I could tell that she was doing things even though she didn't feel good. She just wanted to spend time with me.

Karen had to leave the Navy for medical reasons. Because of her heart issues, she couldn't pass the physical. Fortunately, she was in aircraft maintenance and was able to get a similar job with United Airlines. She was a maintenance supervisor for United. Part of her job was making sure planes all over the country, and maybe all over the world, had their parts. She did that for almost two years until she passed away.

I was traveling on the road with Rawlings when Karen died. I was in Durham, North Carolina visiting the Durham Bulls. We were in town for the weekend and were putting on a show at the stadium. I remember that weekend being at the hotel and getting the call.

I talked to my mom every Sunday night. After that, I would call Mike Redohl. When I got off the phone with my mom, I called Mike and was talking to him on

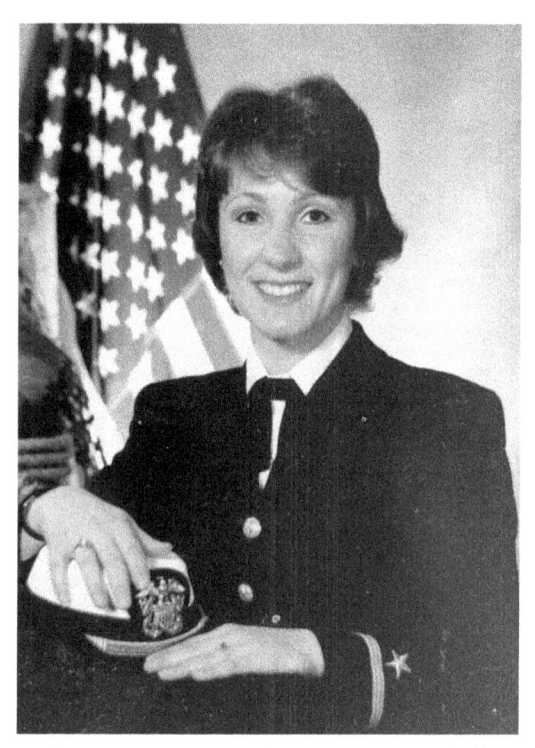

Jim's sister Karen

the phone when I heard a voice in the background, another neighbor who is very close to my mom. "Do you have Jimmy on the phone?" she asks as she enters the room. "I've got to talk to Jimmy."

She picked up the phone and told me, "Jimmy, I'm so sorry to have to tell you this, but Karen has passed away." I was just kind of speechless. We knew that Karen was sick at the time. We knew she had health problems. But it's still a shock when it happens.

That started off a very long night. I had to get to the airport the next morning. My partner that I worked with on the Rawlings Sports Caravan took me in the cab of the truck the next morning. We started out about 6:30, but we actually drove to the wrong airport. They didn't have my flight there, so I realized my flight was at a different airport. Fortunately, it was less than an hour away.

We got there in time, I had my things, flew home, and I think it was around 1 in the afternoon when I got home. Then I was on a 4 o'clock flight to San Francisco. I was on a big plane and there were seats in the back, so I just moved to the back of the plane so I could be alone. I just cried the whole way out there. When the plane landed, I remember a very kind stewardess coming up to me and saying, "I'm so sorry, sir. I hope everything works out OK." She didn't even know what had happened.

Some of Karen's friends met me at the airport. We went to one of the United terminals where they had a memorial celebration for her. It was a touching moment. I got to speak to people who worked with her. I became very close with those people.

I was on the plane home with Karen's casket in less than 48 hours. I remember we flew through Denver and they transferred the casket from one plane to the next. I remember going out on the tarmac and seeing the transfer take place. It was a military transfer, and I was certainly proud of that.

About two weeks before Karen passed, she was at home for my brother Bill's wedding. She had told me that she wasn't doing very well. I think she was really struggling at that time. As a matter of fact, when she passed, Bill and his wife were on their honeymoon in Hawaii. We decided to let them come home before we told them, so my sister Laura went to the airport to pick them up. When they got back to the house, I was the one to tell them Karen had passed. It was tough.

When Karen passed, obviously I was very sad. But my first thought was she could have survived. I certainly hope she got the care she needed. It was really hard for me to understand.

I remember Karen being young, vibrant and beautiful. I was the guy who got a lot of accolades in the family. I was the guy who was achieving things in sports. I was getting the attention, but she was the hero in the family. She went on and on and fought through all this adversity. She was my hero.

The Earthquake Series

Not long after Karen passed, I was back on the road with Rawlings. I went to California for the World Series between San Francisco and Oakland, the Battle of the Bay series that became known as the Earthquake Series. I was at the game at Candlestick Park in October of '89 when the earthquake hit. We had the caravan truck parked out in the parking lot, and I was in the museum trailer at the time the earthquake hit.

I didn't know what had happened. I thought another truck hit us because the museum was shaking. I remember poking my head out the door of the truck and it was still rocking a little bit. I came down the stairs and immediately noticed people running through the parking lot with their kids. I stopped one gentleman and said, "What are you doing?" He said, "We just had an earthquake. I'm getting to my car."

That scared me because if you have a local guy really scared, this must have been something really big. We just stayed put for a very long time. In fact, we had a generator on our truck, and a lot of the news media came over to the caravan to plug their units in and do what they needed to do to get their stories out.

Finally, we left at about midnight. Because of damage to the bay bridge, we drove south to San Jose, took a short bridge and went back around San Francisco all the way back to our hotel in Oakland. I don't think we got back to the hotel until about 1:30 in the morning. It was a long day.

It was a very hard time for me because Karen just died earlier that year. My mom was absolutely petrified that I was in San Francisco. We knew the guys in the ABC truck, so before we left the stadium parking lot that night, I was able to call my mom from their truck to let her know that I was OK. I knew she would have been devastated if something had happened to me.

Chapter 8

Julie

The sports caravan didn't travel after the World Series, so I was home for a while. One night my friend Dominic Barczewski and I were at my house watching a Blues hockey game. When the game was over, I actually said, "I'm going to bed." Dom was like, "no, no, we're going out." I didn't feel like going out. But we did.

There was a restaurant down on Southwest Avenue — Harry's Bar and Grill — down there by Southwest Bank. It was kind of a popular place at the time. A guy from Oakville, Mike Thone, owned the place, and a couple of his friends from Oakville worked down there.

We met two girls down there that night. One of them we knew, Maria Traina. Her brother was a big soccer player, Nick Traina (*he and Dom were teammates for a year at UMSL*). So Nick's sister was good friends — in fact, they were roommates — with this other girl, Julie Crespi. I talked to her that night and eventually asked her out.

I remember our first date. We played tennis at Suson Park and I could tell right away that she was extremely athletic. She was 5-9, slender, but strong. I spent some time before that day researching her background because I wanted to know more about her. She played volleyball and tennis in college at UMSL and then played volleyball at Rockhurst. Playing tennis with her and seeing her play volleyball, I could tell that she was very competitive… and a very good athlete. I actually thought she had better athletic skills and ability than I did.

I don't remember us keeping score, but I think I won the match on our first date. I knew I was competitive, but she was really competitive, maybe more than me. I just kept thinking to myself, "man, if I marry this girl and we have babies, they'll be amazing athletes."

Julie comes from a very athletic family. Her uncle — Frank "Creepy" Crespi — played on the Cardinals team that won the World Series in '42. He was a very good player, but he injured his leg in the war and never made it back to the big leagues. Julie's brother, Tom, was a very good athlete, too. He was a very good volleyball player and a competitive long-distance biker.

Julie was playing almost every weekend in these club volleyball tournaments. Julie would leave at 6 or 7 in the morning on a weekend and she wouldn't get back till about 8 or 9 at night. Then she would do the same thing the very next day.

I remember the first time I went to see her play. I didn't know what to expect. She was playing front row at the time and she would just get up in there, hang there, and just power the ball, spiking it to the floor. My eyes were just wide open because I knew I couldn't hang like that.

I also remember going on a trip with Julie to Florida in the spring of '91. She wanted to see her sister in Orlando, but that was about five hours away from where we were staying. I told her I didn't feel like driving. I just wanted to relax. The next thing you know we're in a rental car driving five hours to Orlando. That's kind of when I realized, "I guess I'll end up marrying this girl."

But actually we had a good time. We went to meet her sister, who had a young daughter, Julie's niece. Julie was very close to her. I remember going to a water park to see a ski show. We had a really good time.

We ended up getting engaged in August of '91. I was getting ready to come off the road for Rawlings that year. We would see each other off and on during that summer. Every chance I would get, I would fly home to see her. I was sort of home for the summer in August when we had a dinner planned at my house.

Julie was very, very late; I think it was because of an all-day volleyball tournament. I was fixing dinner — it wasn't anything special — but she finally got to my house and that's when I proposed. That's the night we got engaged.

It was more than sports that attracted me to Julie. She was not all about herself, just a nice Catholic girl from a great family. I loved her smile and loved more than anything to see her laugh, and you know, we just had fun together. We were who we were and didn't have to pretend. We just really enjoyed each other, and it became very evident because we were always together.

Chapter 9

Slowing Down

In October of 1991 we (*my fiance Julie and myself*) went to the OktoberFest in Hermann, Missouri with my good friend Mike McCartney and his girlfriend. We took an Amtrak train from the Kirkwood station to Hermann and spent the day there. I remember walking up a hill to the Stone Hill Winery, which is a pretty big hill and a long walk. As we're walking, every 10 to 15 feet, I had to stop. I knew something wasn't right. I couldn't get my breath. Here I am, an ex-pro athlete, I shouldn't have to stop like that.

I knew when I got home that I had to go to the doctor. I remember my mom and myself going to the doctor initially at St. Anthony's Hospital. He ordered some tests — a cardio echogram. I remember waiting in the waiting room for him to come out. He told us what was going on. "It looks like you have cardiomyopathy," he said.

The doctor said they didn't know what kind it was, idiopathic or it could be viral. A viral cardiomyopathy is a virus, which there was always a possibility it could go away. But the chances of that were not great given the past record of my family. My sister had already passed, my father passed, so we assumed it wasn't viral.

I had a tearful session with my mom. My mom just did as she always did. "OK, Jimmy, you know you can do this," she said. I remember the doctor at St. Anthony's saying, "If you need a new pump, we'll get you a new pump. There are doctors in St. Louis that can do that, both at St. Louis U. and Barnes. We'll get you a new pump."

Getting to Barnes

I became more aware of Barnes Hospital and decided I wanted to try to get to Barnes. I thought that was the best place in St. Louis to get treatment, prepare for surgery and get on the transplant list. That winter I went on a trip for Rawlings to a trade show in Atlanta; it was the biggest trade show of the year. I was really scared going on the trip because I had a lot of swelling in my ankles. After the show ended each day, I would walk back to the hotel. It was always a slight incline walking back. It was tough for me. I had to rest.

One day while I was in Atlanta I got a hold of the nurse transplant coordinator at Barnes (*her name was Cindy Behrends, now Cindy Pasque*). She took a very long time to talk with me and explain the process of getting me into Barnes and officially start seeing the people there, which I'm glad because I had this fear I was going to die in Atlanta. That could have happened.

Cindy sort of became my lifeline. She took me under her wing, treated me like I was her brother, and made sure that I got everything I needed at Barnes. I got back from Atlanta, finally got down to Barnes and started seeing the docs down there. The first doctor I saw was a guy named Dr. Craig Reiss. Craig was considered one of the young guns at Barnes. These are the guys you want to be your doctors. There were probably three to five of them down there at the time — and he was one of

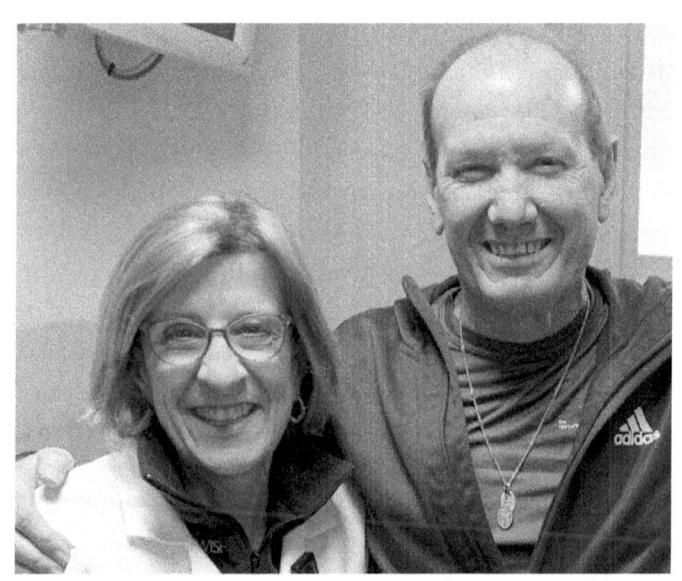

Jim with Cindy Pasque

them. He was not a surgeon; he was a cardiologist. These are the guys that keep you going until it's time for surgery.

The first time I met Dr. Reiss was very interesting. I could tell right away that he was very soft-spoken with a good bedside manner. I just felt like this guy wasn't going to let me die, and dying was a very real possibility. So I went down to see him on a Tuesday or Wednesday. I left that day with a Holter monitor; that's a monitor they put on you for 24 hours to monitor your heart rhythm during that entire 24-hour period. I think it was a Thursday that I came back and turned the monitor in, and then they checked the results on Friday.

"I'm Looking for Jim Tietjens"

I was due to go to a wedding rehearsal dinner that night with Julie; it was down at the Cupples House at St. Louis University. When Dr. Reiss saw the results from the Holter monitor, I had consistent episodes of what they call V-Tach (*ventricular tachycardia*). V-Tach is a kind of abnormal heartbeat that can kill you instantly. Your heart is in chaos and nothing is working together. I would have episodes from 1,200 to 2,400 of those without getting back into normal rhythm. That was really unheard of, to have that number and still be alive.

When Dr. Reiss saw those readings, it was probably late in the day. In my mind, he was like, "We have to find this guy. We have to find him right away." He remembered that his nurse coordinator was friends with Maria Traina. I told him that my fiance lived with Maria. His nurse coordinator was able to get a hold of Maria that same day. They knew the situation was urgent, so they found an invitation for the rehearsal dinner I was supposed to attend in the trash can at their house. They got the address and location of the dinner.

I was at the rehearsal dinner fairly late (*it was about 10 o'clock*). I was struggling. I was tired and wanting to get home, so I went to the lobby to get my coat and Julie's coat. At the time, I was there by myself, no one was with me. And then the door opens… it's a policeman. When he walked in the door, I knew he was looking for me. "He says, "I'm looking for Jim Tietjens." I very calmly said, "that's me." He said, "you need to call this number right away." It was the number for Dr. Reiss.

So I called Dr. Reiss. He says, "Jim, I want you to go to the hospital right now." I told him I was at the Cupples House and then asked if I could go home and put some things in a bag. He said, "No. I want you to stop what you are doing, get in the car, and get to the hospital right now."

So I walk back to my fiance, bring her coat, and tell her that I need to go to the hospital right now. She kind of thought I was joking around, but I said, "No, I'm serious." All of a sudden, most of the dinner party — it was about 16 to 20 people at the most — came down to the hospital with me. I got to the hospital and went right up to a room. Immediately, I took off all my clothes and they got a gown on me. They were afraid an episode could happen to me at any time. We went from eating cake, having drinks, having a nice dinner, to "Jim's in the hospital in ICU."

That was my first hospitalization. It was in December of '91 and I was in the hospital for at least seven to 10 days. They were seeing if I was swelling, checking my heartbeat, and getting me on the necessary meds to try to calm that rhythm down. So now we get to the point where Dr. Reiss feels good about sending me home. At that time, my ejection fraction was 30 percent. Normally it would be 50 to 75 percent; that's a normal ejection fraction. It's showing the pumping power of the heart muscle. It's not the only thing telling you if the heart is sick or not, but it's telling you if the heart is pumping decent enough.

Making the Transplant List

Cindy had set up Dr. Reiss with my heart team. They agreed it was time to see them. My hope was that the heart transplant would be coming soon. You know, a lot of people don't live long enough to get one. Things weren't getting better for me; things were getting worse. Dr. Reiss was trying to keep me stable as long as he could.

On February 25 — that's my birthday — that's when I got on the transplant list. I was in and out of the hospital for the next few months. They make sure you're not going anywhere until you're stable.

Julie moved in with me soon after that, and they set up CPR training for people in my family. We had a meeting with the doctors, my parents and Julie's parents. Both of our parents were pretty much against us living together before we were married, so we met with the doctors and her priest and got them to sign off on it so that the moms and dads were comfortable with the situation.

Getting Married

Julie and I got married on May 9 at St. Gabriel Catholic Church. Julie grew up there, she went to St. Gabriels, it was a beautiful church. We had known the priest there — Father Burgoon — we met him when we were engaged, so I was very comfortable with that church. And, obviously, I wanted Julie to be happy.

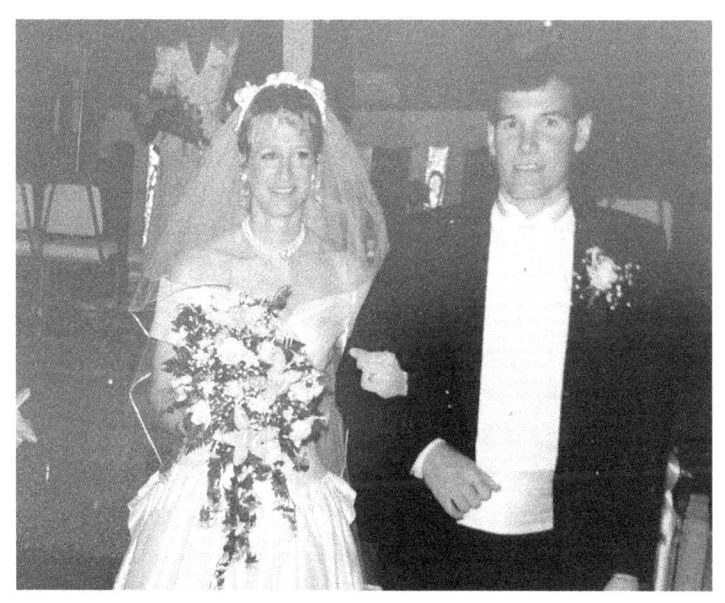

Jim's wedding day

We talked to Dr. Reiss about whether we should postpone the wedding. Is the wedding going to cause me more stress? If we called it off, would that cause me more stress? We decided to go ahead with the wedding. I actually was in a chair up at the altar. I really tried to talk Julie out of marrying me at that time because I had seen what happened in my family. I wasn't sure if we would be able to have kids, and I really tried hard to convince her that "hey, we can do this later." But she wouldn't have any part of it. She loved me. I loved her. It really says a lot about her. She gave me so much support at the time. Julie believed in me. She believed that I could get through anything, so we went on with the wedding.

A couple of things stand out from the wedding. I was a friend of Tom Pagnozzi, the catcher for the Cardinals, because of my job at Rawlings. Tom was at the wedding that day with his wife. The reception followed the wedding at like 12 or 1. He was at the reception with his wife, but they had to leave early because the Cardinals had a game that night.

So that night the Cardinals were getting killed — they were losing 9-0 to the Atlanta Braves. Julie and I were in our room at the Radisson Hotel in Clayton. It had a jacuzzi in the room. We were both tired. She was sleeping on the bed and I had my legs in the jacuzzi because my doctors did not want me to get in there all the way. I'm watching the game and the Cardinals are making a comeback. The Cardinals end up winning the game, 12-11.

The very next night the Cardinals came back again to beat the Braves, and Pagnozzi got the winning hit in the bottom of the ninth. Later that summer during an interview on the radio he said to Jack Buck, "I'm thinking of my friend Jim Tietjens, who is in the hospital at Barnes, and want to offer him prayers for a speedy recovery."

After we got married, we had this journey in and out of the hospital. Julie would drive me down there for therapy and stuff. Now it's summer, I get to the hospital and the doctor says, "you're here to stay. You're not going anywhere." That was music to my ears because there was talk earlier about them putting a defibrillator inside my chest (*the purpose would be to zap my heart automatically if I went into one of those bad heart rhythms*). I didn't want to do that because the defibrillator was a pretty big surgery. Joe Rogers, who was the medical director of our cardiac team, and Dr. Reiss agreed with that decision.

Julie would come to the hospital every day. I had a corner room in Queens Tower. It was my own room, like a suite. I would sit in the window sill every day and look for her car. She would go to work and then come to the hospital after work. I would wait for her car to make the turn into the parking lot and come up to Barnes because I just wanted to see her. My dream was to be a husband, a father and a grandfather. I always felt more comfortable when she was around. It just made me fight through my health challenges.

There was one scary moment that I remember, though, when Julie wasn't there. I was in the hospital waiting for my new heart when I had V-Tach. My room was all the way down at the end of the hall away from the nurses station. I was sitting on the edge of the bed and I felt dizzy. All of a sudden I hear a stampede of people running down to my room. There's like five or six people there, nurses, doctors, my cardiologist, Dr. Reiss.

As soon as Dr. Reiss got in the room, he pushed me gently down to the bed. The docs have their stethoscopes and they're all listening to my heart. Some were pounding on my chest to get my heart out of its bad rhythm. They gave me some medicine to calm me down, and I began to black out. I thought I might have been dying.

"We Have a Heart For You"

I remember the week I got a call from my transplant team. I knew something was going on because it was like dinner time, around 5 o'clock, and they weren't serving me dinner. My nurse that day — I'll never forget her name — was Marissa. I was waiting for dinner because I was hungry and I saw the nurses bringing the trays around. Marissa was in the room and I said, "where's my dinner? I'm supposed to get chicken fingers."

Marissa was kind of quiet and shy and she looked at me and said, "Jim, you're not going to be eating tonight." Right away, I knew. I said, "Marissa, don't tease me." She said, "I'm not teasing you." There were still a lot of checks and balances, but that's when I knew I was about to get the transplant. We may have an offer for Mr. Tietjens tonight — that's how it was presented.

There's a lot of tests going on with the heart. It turned out the donor was the result of a head injury, a motorcycle accident. The doctors at Barnes are ordering tests to see if there was trauma to the heart and just making sure the heart is healthy. Did this young person have any heart issues? How fast can the heart come out of the body? How soon can surgery be done? The last thing is the surgeons have to visibly see the heart.

Fortunately, Julie's sister, niece and nephew were in town from Florida. They told me they were going out to eat that night at a restaurant on Hampton, a great Italian place. I called the restaurant and explained the situation. I talked to her on the phone and told her that it looked like I would be getting the transplant, but there was no need to rush to the hospital. I think she got there later that night like around 9, 10 o'clock, which was fine.

I actually fluctuated between Numbers 1 and 2 on the transplant list. There was another man, Phil, who was very sick and needed a heart real bad. We were in the hospital together and became friends. I would go over to his room and he would come over to mine. We would talk; he was just a wonderful man.

Phil talked his doctors into letting him go home that Fourth of July weekend. I became No.1 on the transplant list because Phil was not in the hospital.

I got the heart.

Chapter 10

First Transplant

People ask me if I was scared the night before my surgery. At that point, I had so much confidence in that hospital. They all took me under their wing and took care of me, even the people who cleaned the room. I was this young man that was going to be a success story and they were going to make sure of it. They weren't going to let anything bad happen to me. So, no, I don't remember being scared.

That night, friends and family came to the hospital. Julie was there. Her sister was in town. As a family, we were all there. My mom was there, my sister Laura was there, my niece, my cousins, my best friend Mike was there. Dom, Gus, Mike McCartney were there. They were all there.

I remember getting in the elevator on the way to the surgery. Everyone gathered around for a prayer. Really the prayer was for someone who just lost his life. As happy as we are right now, there's a family that's really suffering. Let's pray to give strength to the family. And bless the surgeons and everyone in the room.

That was it. The doors closed and I was on my way down to surgery. Once you get down there in the operating room, it all happens so quick. I didn't have time to be nervous. I said to myself, "Let's go, Jim. Let's do it."

When I woke up from the surgery, the first 48 hours were really tough because my kidneys were not working as they should. When you get a new organ, you're being dosed with a lot of medicine. Some of that medicine can affect different organs, and my kidneys were one of them.

They kept me in ICU (*Intensive Care*) for two to three days, and I remember not feeling good. When your kidneys don't feel well, you don't feel well. I remember opening my eyes and the doctor telling me the heart is doing very well. They put it in and it started beating right away. The kidneys aren't doing great, but that's not uncommon. Give them a few days.

When I got out of surgery, my kidneys didn't go back to normal. During the whole time of transplantation, they would probably consider me in minor kidney failure. The kidneys were slowly going bad from the heart medication. I would feel it. I wasn't 100 percent, but it wasn't going to stop me from recovering.

After about three days, Dr. Michael Pasque — he was the head surgeon — brought a stationary bike into my room. My first thought was, "holy cow, are you nuts?" I had this fear of things just stretching, the stitches snapping and blood shooting all over the place. He said "no, you've got a good heart, you're athletic, I want you on this now."

I got on it and felt pretty good. Every day I was a little more confident in myself. For a doctor to walk in on the fourth day following surgery and put a stationary bike in my room, that was pretty incredible.

My heart was performing great, but my issues were with how my kidneys were performing. I was in the hospital for about 10 days so they could get my kidney function back down to normal. They had a lot to balance with a new heart in the body — balance the blood pressure, the pulse, make sure everything is working together.

I finally started getting better. One night the following weekend was sort of an anniversary for me and Julie. I forget what it was, but we were going to eat and celebrate. On the 14th floor of the hospital, they had a restaurant. Julie came to the hospital in a dress and we were going to eat in the restaurant.

So we walked up to the restaurant... and it was closed. She was kind of sad because it was our chance to go out. I started thinking, "well, they said we could go out to dinner. Why don't we just take a ride to The Hill and we'll just be really careful."

I had this male nurse that night. I asked him if he could keep my IV in and take out the cord because I said I was going to be walking and exercising in the stairwell. He said, "yeah, we can do that." I asked if my wife and I could go outside and get some fresh air. "Yeah, no problem," he answered.

I said to Julie, "you go get the car. I'll meet you out front." So Julie gets the car, we're at Kingshighway, you can get to The Hill pretty quick from there. We went to a restaurant. I ate light because I wanted to have a heart healthy meal, so I asked for a light pasta sauce, low sodium, just mostaccioli, no cheese.

I remember every bump in the car on the ride back to the hospital. We eventually got back to my room and didn't do any damage. We probably shouldn't have done it, but I was young and we were in love, so that turned out to be a fun night. You just do things when you are younger. I wanted to do this for her.

Before I was released from the hospital, I asked the doctors when I could have sex. They said you can't have sex until you walk up and down the stairs with a gallon of milk. So, that day Julie's driving me home, we get in the house, I go to the refrigerator, I open the door to the basement, I walk down the stairs, I walk up the stairs, and I said, "OK, let's go."

Cardiac Therapy

About four weeks after the transplant, I came down with a virus. I got something called CMV, the cytomegalovirus. I was brought to the hospital quickly and this amazing physician, Dr. Joseph Kenzora, looked at a cardio echogram and said my heart was fine. However, I had a 105-degree fever. I think my mom stayed the night, icing me up all night to keep my temperature down. I had to have intravenous medicine at home. I would say that was a semi-serious incident.

I enrolled in a cardiac therapy program at St. Anthony's. I toured the place and saw that they had an amazing facility. They were great there. I was there getting monitored every day. I would do the bike, rowing machine, treadmill, and light weights. I did it for at least five months. When it was time to get released, it gave me complete confidence to be out there on my own.

There are a lot of side effects to going through a transplant because your body is blasted with these high doses of heart medication, like prednisone and other immunosuppressive drugs. They kind of give you the shakes, make your ankles swell up a little bit. But the more you exercise, the more you offset the side effects.

If I wouldn't be at the gym, honestly, that's what is keeping me alive. If I would stay at home and just eat snacks every day, I would be in trouble. It's just not in my DNA. It's also about the gifts I have been given. I feel I'm in debt to not only repay my donor but his mother, his father, those people, too.

I was pretty happy with my recovery. I do things only one way, and that's to attack it. I'm pretty good at recovering from injuries and things like that. I don't look at it as an obstacle. I look at it as a challenge.

Time Off From Rawlings

After the heart transplant, Rawlings was nice enough to give me six months off. Julie and I took advantage of that time to do some traveling. We went on a cruise to Grand Cayman and Jamaica, which was wonderful. We went to Fort Lauderdale, we went to the Florida Keys. That was our first real time together as a married couple, like a honeymoon. We just had a really good time.

When we went on the cruise, the doctors told me to be careful about scuba diving because of the (*water*) pressure, so I didn't snorkel. I introduced myself to the ship doctor just to let him know what was going on with me, but there never was a need for him. They had a gym on the ship and I was in it early every morning. Julie wasn't always pleased with that.

We went to Florida at Thanksgiving. Dr. Kanell, the doctor who did my knee surgeries, had us over for Thanksgiving dinner. I was so proud to have her meet them. They were just amazing people.

We tried to do a lot here in St. Louis too. We went to the Lake of the Ozarks a lot because we had a boat. We would go to the lake with friends, her friends and sometimes my friends, and we would have a good time there.

Overall, it was six months that we really tried to enjoy. And we did.

Chapter 11

Back To Work

Not long after I started back to work at Rawlings I had become aware of the World Transplant Games. The '93 Games were held that year in Vancouver, British Columbia. I did a lot of running post-transplant, doing a lot of sprints, things like that, and my body was OK. But, honestly, six months was not enough to prepare my body for something like this.

Still, I thought to myself, "Hey, I'm an athlete. I can do this. C'mon, what kind of athletes are going to be up there?" So I got the doctor's release and signed up for the games. I got some sponsors — Anheuser-Busch helped me out, and O'Doul's non-alcoholic beer gave me a bunch of shirts and shorts to wear.

I flew up to Vancouver with Julie and my mom. We went over to register for the events. I registered for tennis and then I signed up for the 100, 200 and 400 races. I've got a new pair of New Balance running shoes, so I'm ready to go. I start walking around checking the place out the first day and I see these guys practicing on the track. They look like Olympians you would see on TV. They all have spikes on, they're all muscular.

The first thing I did was tennis. The rumor was there was a guy in the group who at one time was ranked in Canada. I could see the guy warming up, and I could see that he had played. Unfortunately, I drew him in the first round. We played points, two sets up to 11 points. He won two straight sets against me, but I remember I took two straight points off of him. When we watched the recording, Julie is providing commentary. "JoAnn, I think Jim just took a point… JoAnn, he took another point." It was just a riot. Needless to say, I didn't move on past the first round.

I thought I could do OK in the running events. I thought I was in shape, but my legs had nothing. I got down on the track in the starting position. I look to my right and all I see are track spikes. I look to my left and I see more spikes. I've got my tennis shoes — my running shoes — and I knew I was in big trouble.

One of the races — I think it was the 200 — I went to the next heat. There were only four runners in that one, and I finished second. As I came around the track, my mom was all excited. "Jimmy, you took second." I was like, "Hey mom, there were only four people in the race. Trust me, I didn't qualify."

I could have done much better, but it was a good time. I still remember marching into the stadium for the opening and closing ceremony. We met some interesting people and there were some really good athletes there.

Returning to Rawlings

I had to ask Rawlings if I could go to the games, and they were nice enough to let me off work. But I got back into work pretty quickly. I started off just working a half day to test out my heart. They put me in my old job that I absolutely loved. I went from selling closeouts, you know, products that are old or defective, to selling what we called premium products.

I would sell products with logos on them, big consumer product companies like Pepsi, Coke, Pizza Hut, True Value Hardware. I sold a million baseballs one year to True Value Hardware. It was a dollar a baseball, so it was a million dollar order. I had some amazing years there doing sales.

I loved my job because it was pretty much my own business. I managed every aspect of it. I managed the budget. I got the customers. I managed the shipping, managed working with companies overseas. It was fun, unique, and I did very well.

One World Cup year I sold over 240,000 soccer balls to Lancome Loreal; they make fragrances and Polo Sport cologne. Back in the day, colognes would offer gifts with purchase — "buy this, you get this soccer ball." Those were big orders and they were important because Polo Sport had a high brand image. Those were also million dollar orders.

I sort of made a name for myself at Rawlings. I was well respected and I loved the people there. I was able to come up with my own ideas, get creative and innovative. I had a lot of autonomy.

Things were good.

Chapter 12

The Kids

When I was in the hospital waiting for my first transplant and suffering from V-Tach, I was scared to death. I told Dr. Reiss, with tears in my eyes, "I just want to be a father." He grabbed my hand and said, "Jim, you will be a father."

About three years after my transplant, my son Jimmy was born. Julie really wanted to have a baby, and so did I. We really didn't think much about what could happen with the bad heart gene. It's on your mind, but we never lived in fear. After Jimmy was born, we waited two years and had our second child, our daughter Annie.

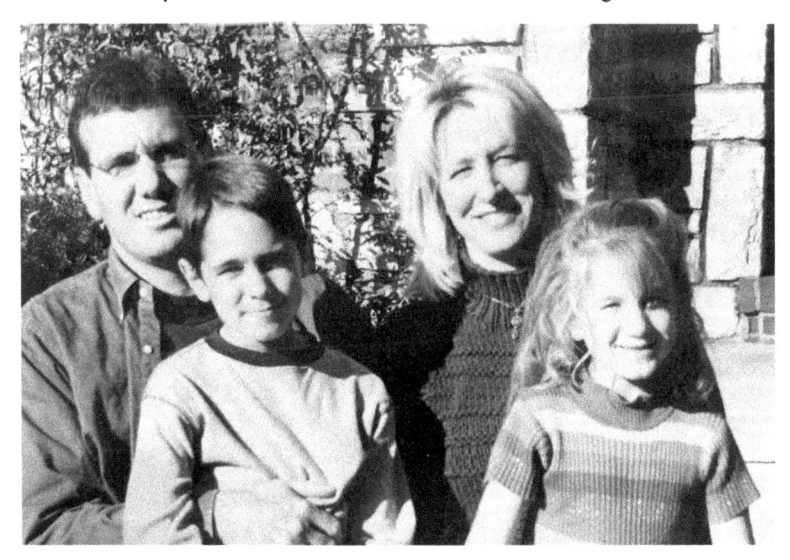

Jim and Julie with kids Jimmy and Annie

Both of my siblings had the bad heart gene, so it was on our minds. My sister Laura had her heart transplant in her early 40s. Her daughter Kortney has already had two heart transplants, and one of Kortney's children is also positive for the bad heart gene.

That has been very difficult for me because both of my children happen to be negative to the bad heart gene. For me, it's a miracle. I remember I was in Ohio at a dialysis center when I got the news about my daughter being negative to the heart gene. Other than the day I got married and the days my kids were born, it was the happiest day of my life.

My son tested negative about four months later. I happened to be in the doctor's office for a biopsy. I told the doctor I had not heard anything about my son's test results. He came back into the room and sort of whispers, "he's negative." When you consider everything that has happened in my family, for my two kids to be negative is completely miraculous. What that means is my daughter, my son, it's gone forever. They don't have the gene and they can't pass it on.

Julie and I were very happy we had two kids. We really did a lot as a family. When I think of the things we did, there were a lot of good times. We were good parents. We tried really hard. We were not perfect, but I think we did a good job.

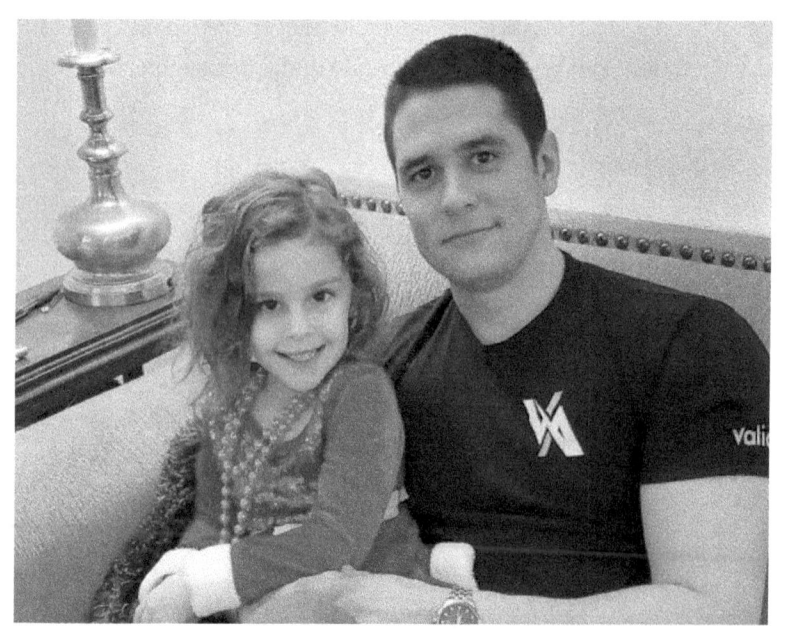

Jimmy with daughter Gia

Jimmy was challenging because he had ADHD (*Attention-deficit/Hyperactivity Disorder*). It was hard for me to understand it. Julie researched it a great deal and learned a lot about it. To a lot of people it can come across as misbehavior, but that is not correct. It has more to do with the ability to focus and concentrate.

Jimmy played baseball, basketball and soccer and was good at all those sports. He was a natural athlete. ADHD made it difficult on him because at some point in the game he would lose his ability to focus. People that did not understand ADHD — including myself — could get very frustrated with him. This frustration at times could turn into anger and at that point nothing good would come of it.

Jimmy has come a very long way and I am so proud of him. He has always excelled in sales roles because of his ability to communicate with people and his competitive spirit. He has matured a great deal and has shown a keen interest in reading.

Jimmy is a great father to his daughter Gia (*born 2014*) and time and time again I am thankful Gia has him as her father.

Along Came Annie

Annie, meanwhile, was born in 1997. From Day One, she was precious. We always thought Annie was going to be a nun because she is so, so sweet. She just loved her brother. If he didn't get enough to eat, she would say, "Jimmy, you can have some of mine. I'll share with you, Jimmy."

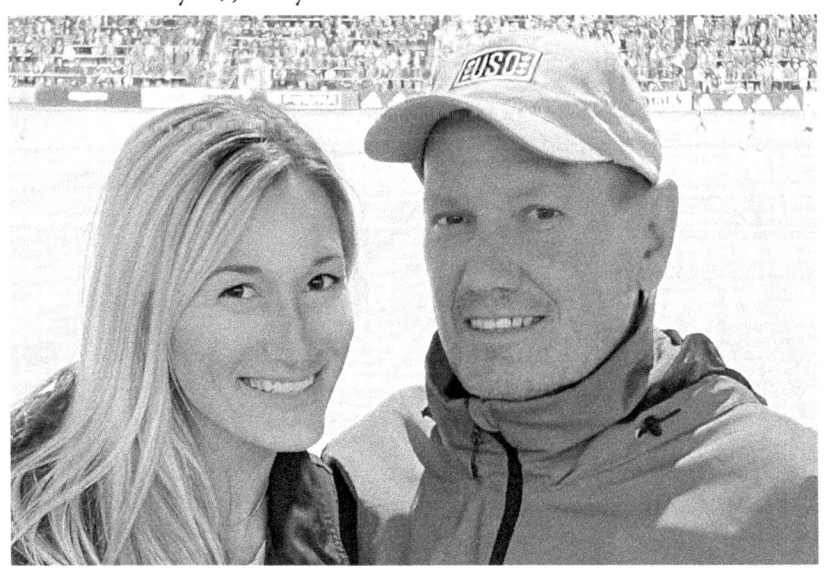

Jim with daughter Annie

Annie was really small when she was a kid, but she would try anything. When Annie went to the park, she would get right up there on the monkey bars. When I first taught Annie how to ride a 2-wheeler, I gave her one push and she was flying. She would do something one time and she got it. She was athletic and she was very brave.

She played volleyball, softball, basketball and soccer growing up. She even played racquetball in high school. Her mom taught her a lot about volleyball working with her one-on-one. Julie was taking all the volleyball responsibility with Annie and I was taking on baseball with Jimmy.

Jimmy played baseball with a traveling team for eight years. He stopped playing when he was a sophomore in high school. It was kind of sad for me because he loved baseball, but it was just too much for him. Some kids get burned out playing 70 games in the summer. That's what he chose, and I respected that.

Annie started playing select volleyball around third grade. Julie did a great job with her. She worked with Annie almost every day in the backyard, just working on her lateral movement and teaching her how to be a setter. On the court, Annie was a gamer and a fighter. She was able to focus, she never had a bad attitude, and she was a leader. I was so proud of how she developed.

Annie went to Ursuline Academy for high school and was an all-stater there. She got an offer for a full-ride scholarship to a Division II school in Ohio. We went up there for a visit, but when we came out of a restaurant on Halloween night, there was a blizzard, snow everywhere. Annie said, "I'm not going here."

So that was a little disappointing. Annie wanted to play Division I, but the big schools were recruiting 6-foot setters, and Annie was only 5-7. She had a few offers from smaller Division I schools, but none of them seemed to be a fit for her. She wanted to play at a school in the south. So she ended up going to a place in Mobile, Alabama called Spring Hill College, a private Catholic Division II school.

Annie had to sit out her first year because she got injured during her club volleyball season her senior year of high school, but then she played her second year. They won a lot of games that year, a couple of tournaments. One weekend Annie went wild and had an unbelievable tournament. Parents in the stands were talking about how well she was playing.

Annie was named the team's MVP that year. She made the all-conference and all-region teams. And she was named the top setter in the conference.

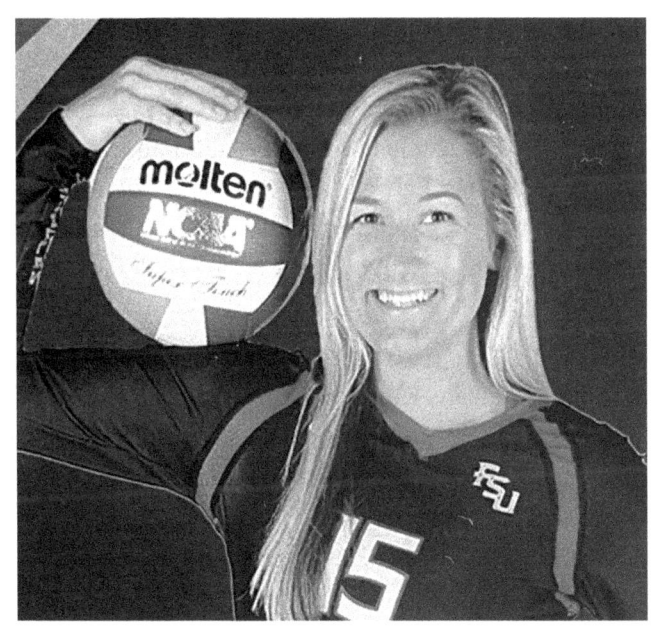

Annie at Florida State

After that season, Annie told her coach that she wanted to play Division I. She had discussions with schools like Georgia, Auburn, Alabama, Tulane, Alabama-Birmingham. She also had been talking to the University of South Alabama, and they had seen her tapes. They had an assistant coach there who graduated from Florida State. Before the season, Florida State signed a 6-1 setter out of Ohio, but she had issues with her knees. The signing period was over. All the top prospects were signed. Florida State needed another setter.

While this was going on, the assistant at South Alabama returned to Florida State as an assistant coach there. This coach talked to the head coach at Florida State and said she had film on Annie. So they looked at the film and brought Annie in as their second setter. I still remember her telling me, "Dad, are you sitting down? Florida State wants to sign me."

Florida State ran a two-setter system, so Annie came in and shared time with the other setter. I was so proud of her. No one thought she could do it because of her lack of athletic physique, but she did it. She hung in there for two years at Florida State.

Annie had one season of eligibility left, but she was pretty much done with school at Florida State. But Indiana wanted her. They offered her a chance to come in and be their setter. She also said that Nebraska offered her a scholarship.

Annie turned down the offers. When I asked her why she didn't take it, she said, "Dad, I'm so beat. I'm so sore… ankles, elbows, knees.. I'm done."

The funny thing is when Annie was growing up, she was always the player the better teams didn't want. But Annie has the mental toughness and the willingness to work to make herself better. I always said that some coach one day is going to realize what Annie can do and he's going to take her. And that's what happened at Florida State.

A Cardiac Nurse

Annie decided to pursue a career in nursing. She graduated No. 1 in her class at the Goldfarb School of Nursing and is now a cardiac ICU nurse at Barnes. She works with some of the same people that worked on me during my transplants. She realizes that without these people, she wouldn't be here.

Annie chose to do this on her own. I'm so proud of her.

Chapter 13

McGwire Mania

After my career with the sports caravan was over, I moved into the offices at Rawlings. I became the close-out sales director, and I did that for a few years. From that I became the Rawlings Premium and Incentive Sales manager, so I was selling custom equipment for promotions.

That was right around the time Mark McGwire set the single-season home run record. I always wanted to try to find new things to do, so when McGwire hit all those home runs in 1998, I came up with an idea to create commemorative Mark McGwire bats. I worked with a couple people here and a couple people in other states to create these bats. Most of the bats sold for over $100 apiece.

We did the commemorative "No. 60" bat when he tied Babe Ruth. When he tied Roger Maris, we did a "61" bat. Then we did a "62" bat when he beat Roger Maris' home run record. And then we did a "70" bat at the end of the season. The cost of the bat to the consumer went up each time he hit a new milestone. Each time I created a bat that was laser engraved with facts on the bat about the home run — the date, the distance of the home run, etc. We even laser engraved his autograph on it.

It was a pretty exciting time. He and Sammy Sosa were going at it as they tried to set the home run record. I told the Rawlings president we could sell these bats, but we need two new laser engraving machines. And we did it.

We did another commemorative bat when Mark hit his 500th career home run in August of '99. After it was all over, we ended up putting another seven figures in Mark's pocket (*and his agent's*). He had a contract to use our bats and gloves, but no

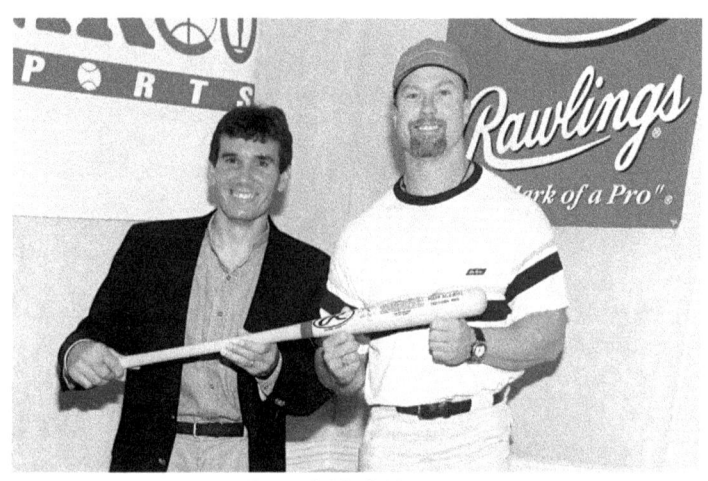

Jim with Mark McGwire

one was making over a hundred grand to do that. Nothing came close to the money we were making off the commemorative bats.

Representing McGwire

I got to know Mark's agent — his name was Jim Milner. He was a great guy and we became close. Jim liked me, and he liked the work that I was doing. At one point he called the president of Rawlings — Howard Keene — and told him he wanted me to handle everything Rawlings does with Mark McGwire. So I became the Rawlings rep for McGwire.

I remember the first day I met Jim. He came to St. Louis on a really hot day in May and I picked him up at the airport. I used to drive an old Chevy S10 Blazer; it was old and pretty beat up. I was kind of like, "I'm just going to drive this until it drops." It's one of those things where, you know, you're younger and you don't worry about whether or not the air conditioning works.

So I go up to the airport, and I had not had the air conditioning on in probably eight months. Jim's a big guy, he's got a navy blue blazer on, a blue dress shirt, and it's hot outside. I pick him up and I'm going to take him down to the ballpark. I tried to turn on the AC and nothing was coming out. The car is jerking forward and I'm thinking, "Man, this is embarrassing." I'm just praying we get down to the stadium.

Somehow we get to the old Busch Stadium and I park on the curb where the player's entrance is located, and I drop him off there. We get out of the car, he looks down, and green antifreeze is coming out underneath my car. So he's making a joke about that and we just moved on.

New Wheels

Later in '98 — I think it was the day after McGwire hit home run No. 62 — I had the flu. But I had to be in the office that day because there was so much going on related to the McGwire stuff. Howard Keene asked me a couple of times that day if I was going to be in the office that afternoon. I told him, "I have to be, even though I'm not feeling well, there's too much going on, so I'll be here."

At 2 o'clock in the afternoon, he calls me into his office. He walks over to the window and he's got a set of car keys in his hand. He says, "Jim Milner called and said, 'Howard, we have to get Tietjens a new car. I'll pay half, you pay half.' I said, 'no, no, Jim, we'll take care of it." So Howard calls me over to the window, looking out at the parking lot, and says, "see that navy blue Blazer? Jim, that navy blue Blazer is yours."

To cap it off, he gave me a gas card… to go along with a brand new four-door navy blue Chevy Blazer. It was nice because my wife and I had a little ski boat and it was nice to pull the boat. It was bigger than what we had. And the air conditioning worked, so that was exciting.

I called my wife and said, "Hey, you're not going to believe this, but I want you to know I just got a new car." She was getting on me because we had agreed not to purchase a new car unless we talked about it. So, I said, "Well, I got a pretty good deal." "What do you mean?" she said. "How much was it?" I said, "Well, it was free. I'll tell you the whole story when I get home."

A Short Vacation

That was quite a week for us. A few days prior to that, my wife and I — and our two young kids — were on vacation in Toronto. We were going to take a train from Canada to Niagara Falls. But things were heating up in St. Louis. Mark had hit home runs 59 and 60 over the weekend, and now the whole country is focused on St. Louis.

It was a Monday night in September and McGwire had just hit No. 61 to tie Maris' record. It's 10 o'clock at night — we're in our hotel room at a Marriott — and I look at my wife and say, "We're getting out of here. The whole baseball world is in St. Louis and we're in Toronto. I'm doing all this stuff with McGwire. Why am I not there?"

There was an airline strike going on in Canada, so we could not get a flight out of Canada. We had a rental car that we had to return in Canada. So we get to the airport about 11:30, midnight. I was there forever exchanging the car for another one that we could take into the U.S.

It was like 1 o'clock in the morning. I saw that we could get a flight out of Cleveland back to St. Louis, so we drove all night to Cleveland. When we got there, the sun was rising. It was a hard night, and I almost fell asleep a couple of times.

We jumped into a Holiday Inn at about 7 a.m. Our flight was at 1 p.m., so we asked the hotel if we could get a room for four hours for like 50 bucks. They said, "sure, sure." My wife and I went to bed, the kids were up the whole time, just running all over the place and jumping on the beds, so we didn't get much sleep.

I called Jim Milner and told him we were going to get into St. Louis around 4:30, 5 o'clock. He said, "I've got you sitting next to the Maris family." I'm thinking, "No, I'm not a big shot at Rawlings. I shouldn't be sitting next to the Maris." So I told Jim, "I can't do that. I can't sit next to them."

So we get into St. Louis, we go home, we got a babysitter for the kids, we literally showered and went down to the ballpark. We were just dead tired. It was a Tuesday night. Steve Trachsel was pitching for the Cubs. And McGwire hits No. 62.

That was an amazing year. I mean, I'm working in baseball. I'm a huge baseball fan. We had a great team. It was just great fun to be part of the McGwire excitement.

Chapter 14

My Dream Job

Rawlings was a special place for me. It was my first real job. It helped me with my business knowledge and allowed me to build my career. I learned how to talk to people in business. When you work on a business deal, it has to be a win-win. If people trust you and like you, that's the biggest thing. Customers knew I could get the job done, and I had the backing of Rawlings to get things done.

However, it has always been my dream to work at Anheuser-Busch. Just driving by there when I was a kid, seeing the Clydesdales at Cardinals games, it was iconic. Many of my best friends worked there — Mike Redohl, Kurt Billmeyer, Mike McCartney. I saw how A-B operated and how they spent money on marketing and promotions, and I wanted to be a part of that. I wanted to prove to my friends that I could cut it there.

I had a successful career at Rawlings, loved the people there, but I felt I was ready to move on. I worked at Rawlings for 13 years, I was 40 years old and figured I better try to do it now. I knew a lot of people at A-B because I sold promotional merchandise to them while working at Rawlings. I had the opportunity to talk to them, I got an interview there, and within a month they offered me a job. This was satisfying to me, but I was a little intimidated. A-B is a giant corporation.

I remember going into the office of the VP of Sales at Rawlings. I was in tears, telling him how much I love Rawlings, how sad I was to be leaving, but that this was a dream of mine. My son Jimmy was a little sad because we got a lot of perks at Rawlings. I always had gloves and gear with his name on it. Every team he was on I got customized Rawlings uniforms. We had equipment supplied for a lifetime —

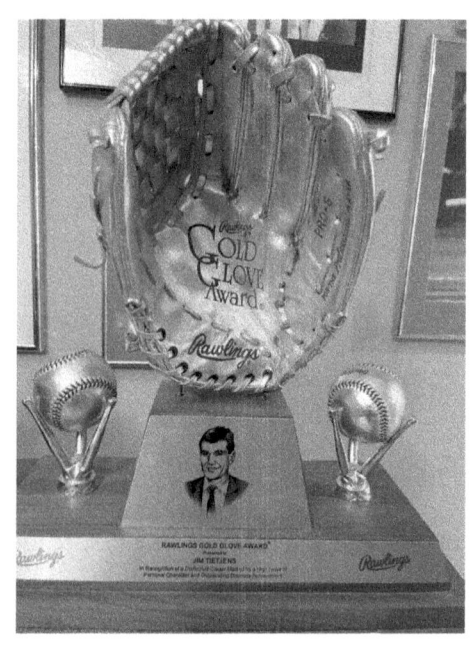

Jim's Gold Glove

gloves, bats, things like that. I told Jimmy, "Don't worry, there will be plenty of perks at A-B."

Our whole family enjoyed Rawlings, we really did. Rawlings ended up presenting me with a Rawlings Gold Glove award, which is pretty impressive. Not just anyone gets that award. It's meant a lot to me over the years.

I remember the day I talked to Howard Keene, a guy I have enormous respect for. I went in personally to tell him I was leaving. At first, he says, "Aw, no, Jimmy, not you…" And then he said, "Never has a finer man walked through those doors." Man, that meant the world to me. Here is this icon of the sporting goods industry telling me that. It was just an incredible compliment from an incredible man.

Transitioning to A-B

I jumped right into the job at A-B. I worked in sales promotions with a team of about eight or nine people. Four or five of us were responsible for working with our frontline sales directors for our biggest accounts in the country. These were supermarket or convenience store accounts — Kroger, Safeway, Albertsons, 7-11, Circle K. The other four of us would be working on promotions for restaurant chains — TGIFridays, Hooters, places like that.

We were very successful, but we also had a lot of fun. The funniest moment came the day after I was painting the bedroom in our house. I was on a big ladder and I was reaching to paint the wall. I was too lazy to get down and move the ladder, and I started sliding off the ladder. My head was on the wall as I'm sliding and it raked the trim around the door.

I knew there was blood coming out because I could feel it. I called for Julie to come in and asked her to call 9-1-1. So she calls the police and the paramedics came. When they got there I was sitting at the bottom of the stairs with a towel on my head. They take me in an ambulance to St. Anthony's Hospital, and they took good care of me there.

I came home from the hospital at 3:30 in the morning. My head is totally wrapped. The accident took the skin and just peeled it away. I was in so much pain that I couldn't sleep.

We had a big meeting the next morning at 8 o'clock. I don't remember what the meeting was about, but I knew I had to be there because I was leading it. It was myself, a couple of guys on my team, and the VP of Sales, Bill Jones. So I go into the office with my head wrapped — and it was always something with me — and they just bust out laughing. I told them the story about what happened and they could not stop laughing.

The guys on my team never let me forget about it. At A-B, we had a Christmas party every year. At the party after that incident, one of the guys on my team — John Quante — came into the party with his head all wrapped up. So that was pretty good.

At A-B, we worked hard. We knew we were selling beer. We were competitive; we wanted to win. But we made sure we had a good time.

Perks of the Job

There were tickets to big events that became available. Occasionally, I was able to have my family in the A-B Suite at Busch Stadium, both the old stadium and the new one. I remember we went to most of the World Series games, whether I had to pay for them myself or not. I was there for the Detroit series (*2006*) and the Rangers series (*2011*).

It had always been a dream of mine to take Jimmy to an all-star game, and I was able to get tickets from our sports marketing department for me and him for the game in Houston in 2004. We also got tickets to a lot of the after-events, so we were able to see up close and personal Roger Clemens, Derek Jeter, and other stars.

One time we were in the same elevator with Hank Aaron. It was myself, Hank Aaron, his bodyguard, and my son. I myself was star-struck, so much so I didn't know what to say. I got out of the elevator and said, "Jimmy, you know who that was?" He said, "No." I said, "Jimmy, that's the greatest home run hitter who ever lived… that's Hank Aaron." He was like, "Aw dad, why didn't you get his autograph?" I said we already have his autograph — on a Rawlings bat.

We had an amazing time in Houston. We got there on a Sunday and flew home Wednesday morning. We had our gloves, father and son out there playing catch, Jimmy wanting to buy every souvenir he saw, all the passes for the different parties, the home run derby. It was a fun time.

I also remember a cool moment at the all-star game in St. Louis in 2009. We were in the upper deck behind home plate and the stealth bomber flew over. There was a lady with two or three little kids sitting three or four rows in front of us. This little kid stands up with a sign, and he was on the scoreboard — "That was our dad." It was unbelievably electric. Here is this little kid honoring his dad and he gets on TV. It was the greatest moment in an all-star game for me.

It was a big moment for us too because Julie's sister was in town for the game. Julie's sister lives in Florida, and for years she had been dating Bob Feller's son, who lives in Orlando. So we went to this pre-game reception to meet Bob Feller, myself and Jimmy, and he signed a ball. You know, Bob Feller was more than just one of the greatest pitchers in the history of the game. He was an American war hero, and more than anything, I respected that.

It was a privilege for me to meet him. It meant a lot to Julie and her family, too.

Chapter 15

Cancer

When I had the first transplant, I was told right away that when you are on immunosuppressive drugs, you have a higher percentage of getting cancer. At the time, I was told it was like 10 to 15 percent greater. What I found out later is that it was more like 30 to 40 percent greater.

It seemed like every January when a new year started, for one reason or another, I did not feel great. The doctor used to think it was more mental than anything. But, this time, as we rolled into 2003, I knew that something wasn't right because I was working myself pretty hard at the gym, I was staying fit in terms of weight and all that stuff, but I couldn't feel myself recovering the next day. I was just dragging.

I remember being at an Anheuser-Busch Christmas party in December of 2002 at the Savvis Center (*now the Enterprise Center*). They had food stations all around the concourse level where you could just walk around the whole thing and get whatever food you wanted. But I just remember I didn't feel well that night. The next day I still didn't feel well. I finally convinced a doctor that something wasn't right and I needed to be checked out.

I would get the night sweats. I would wake up in the middle of the night just sopping wet. That kind of told the doctors that something wasn't normal. They started doing tests on me. Eventually, I saw the infectious disease people and they sent me to a cancer doctor. They isolated something around my stomach area and were getting ready to do a pretty extensive surgery. They had me on a table and would take a lot of scans. They would look at it, come back in the room and take another one. This went on for a couple hours. I was getting really annoyed.

The doctor I was seeing, Dr. Nancy Bartlett — she was an oncologist — came back into the room and was like, "Well, I've got some good news and I've got some bad news." When you're dealing with cancer, you don't want to hear anything about bad news. She said, "the good news is we don't have to do the surgery… but I do believe you have Non-Hodgkin's Lymphoma."

They did a little more detail work on that and came to the conclusion that I had Stage 4 Non-Hodgkin's Lymphoma, which is pretty serious. That was right after the first of the year, and I actually started my cancer treatment in February. They put me on a protocol where I would be getting four different types of chemotherapy.

I had to do 10 months of treatments, two treatments a month. Really, chemo is poison. The doctors try to find the right mix of poison to kill the cancer cells. Fortunately, Barnes was very good at this. I went with Dr. Bartlett, and she would just tell it like it is. Right off the bat, she gave me a 50/50 chance of surviving. I just kind of smiled and said, "I'm going to make it 75/25 because you don't know me, you don't know how I recover, you don't know how I fight. I'm going to give myself those odds."

So we went into the cancer treatment at the Siteman Center. You would be hooked up for four hours getting your four different types of chemo. They wouldn't all come at the same time; they were timed. I remember a lot of chemo I would get on a Wednesday and by Friday I was just totally shot. It was like a truck hit me.

The hope is that you start recovering by the following Tuesday or Wednesday. You had a pause, but every two weeks, you would be back in for more treatment. Some things would delay your treatment. If the white cell count didn't come back to where it needs to be, they couldn't do your chemo. So you would have to get blood transfusions. Of the 10 or 12 treatments I had, I had at least six blood transfusions.

They started re-scanning me after the first three chemo treatments. The chemo was working right away, so mentally that was a real boost for me. Then, after six, it was working really well. The doctor even told me in a quiet way, "I kind of consider you to be in remission."

That was six treatments in and we still had six more to go. At that time I got very sick and they weren't sure exactly what was wrong with me. I began to have this fever; it would be mid-grade during the day and high-grade at night. I would have a 103 or 104 fever at night; they were bad.

Finally, they determined that one of the chemo drugs was damaging my lungs in a pretty big way. So they tested my lungs almost every week. It got to the point where I was stable and I started getting over the fevers. But every time I went in for a lung test, they kept telling me that my lungs had not improved. They said they would finish all the treatments, but they would not give me the one treatment that's hurting my lungs.

I got frustrated because I felt I was getting stronger, but it wasn't showing on the lung test. They kept testing me right up until my last treatment when I got out of the hospital in October. When I got out, I went to the Workout Company. I remember getting on the bike, the pulldown machine. I would do a little exercise every day and I could tell that I was getting stronger.

My next appointment to have a lung test was in November and then I was supposed to come back in December. In November, they said, "we don't see much improvement." I just said, "Listen, you can say whatever you want, but I'm at the gym every day. I know my body, and it's getting stronger."

Sometime before Christmas I went back in for another lung test, and they couldn't believe it. They told me, "Your lungs have healed." I just told them "I told you guys I was getting better, but nobody believed me. You gotta give me credit. I know what I'm talking about. I know my body more than anything."

Fighting cancer was the hardest thing I've ever done in my life. You just have to say you're in this fight for 8 to 10 months, it's not going to be easy, you're going to lose a lot of days, you're going to feel horrible a lot of days, but just try to win one week at a time. That's how I looked at it.

Julie was amazing during that time. She would come with me to every treatment. After the treatment, if I was in good shape, we would go to The Hill and eat. In the treatment center, they have so many amazing snacks — Oreos, Cheetos, the kind of stuff you would put in your kid's lunch. Julie would fill her purse and our bag with those snacks, everything you shouldn't have, but we were eating them.

Jimmy and Annie were very young at the time. They were both attending school at St. Margaret Mary. When I was in the hospital, Julie had to do pretty much everything. I remember, though, when I was home. I would go outside and wait for the kids to walk home together from school. I couldn't walk down the street, so I waited for them to walk up the street. I would get down on my knee to be right at their level so I could give them a hug. I was in tears.

When it was over, I started becoming a real person again. The doctors said my lungs looked great. I knew I was back. I made the 3-year mark cancer free, which is a great position to be in. I was going back every year to get checked. I then made it to the 5-year mark. Dr. Bartlett said right away, "Jim, I consider you cancer free."

A-B was phenomenal during that year. I did not have to worry about one thing. I didn't have to go on disability, always received 100 percent pay, we didn't have to worry about that. I probably went back to work around the beginning of 2004.

Another Cancer Scare

Around 2013, I had this pain under my tongue. I didn't know what it was. I had gone to my dentist and told him I couldn't reach it to see what it was. He looked at it and said I had something that I needed to get looked at, so he sent me to an ear, nose and throat doctor. This doctor looked at it and told me right away, "Jim, it's cancer, but we're going to be able to deal with this."

He told me that this would not be like what I had before, and that gave me a great deal of confidence. He told me it would be like an hour to an hour and a half surgery. I came in for surgery at like 8 or 9 in the morning. I remember being in recovery around 6 that night. When I woke up, I looked at the clock and thought, "Wait a minute, it's 6 o'clock." The doctor came in and said, "Well, it took a little longer than we expected. When we went in, we saw some things we decided to remove. We removed 23 lymph nodes."

In the days after the surgery, I couldn't eat. All I had was liquids, and I lost like 17 pounds. It was hard to even sip anything. They decided there would be no further treatment. They were concerned that I would have developed cancer, so they took all those lymph nodes out. If they had seen cancer, I would have had to follow up with radiation, which never happened.

I couldn't believe how quickly I lost 17 pounds. It was like a week. I have a pair of shorts that I still wear — they're still big on me. At the time they were like 4 inches too big. I remember wearing them to a volleyball party for Annie. I was healthy at that point, but I didn't have any clothes that fit. Annie was chasing me around the yard, and I was running as fast as I could. My pants came down around my butt. That was a little embarrassing.

It was no more than a month, month and a half, though, before I got back to normal.

Chapter 16

Marital Trouble

By the time I reached age 50, I began to slow down again. I had an annual review of my heart, and by 2012 I started getting stents put in. At first, they put two in. A few months later, they put three more in. My ejection fraction slowly began dropping. I could feel myself at the gym losing pace on the treadmill, losing pace on the elliptical. I kind of knew what was coming. I would need a new heart and a new kidney in the next few years.

Because my kidneys were getting worse, I started getting kidney dialysis in 2016. To make things worse, my marriage was not going well. About the time I turned 50 we just started growing apart. Julie started off by sleeping in a different room. She slept upstairs, I slept downstairs. Everything we did was going in different directions. I would go to work, come home, and that was it.

Julie was someone who liked to get out and be social. I was sort of the opposite, especially with my health beginning to fail. She would go out a lot on Thursdays or on the weekend. There were times when I would be home by myself. That didn't sit well with me, but she wanted to get out and be with her friends. It seemed like her friends were becoming a bigger priority than me.

We also had challenges with how we raised the kids, I think more specifically Jimmy, because of his ADHD. We saw multiple doctors and everyone you go to has a different opinion. They'll prescribe different meds. Some work, some don't. You don't know about the damage they might do to him. We would have arguments that sometimes got heated. I thought Jimmy was misbehaving. But Julie was more patient. She had a better feel for how to deal with him than I did. That was my fault.

But that puts a lot of strain on a marriage, especially if you have different ways of looking at things.

We had gone to counseling several times and it seemed all the counseling just made us argue more. One time we were coming down the elevator after a counseling session — and we just had a horrible argument… because the counselor was sort of promoting that — we both looked at ourselves in the elevator and started laughing. "Why are we doing this? What a waste of time — and money."

Julie moved out on November 13, 2017. We had a pretty heated argument. I said, "I know you don't want to be here. You're not happy, so why don't you just leave." And she did. It was a hard time. It was a sad time. I was as much a part of the problem as she was. I wish I would have done better.

The Good Times

I'm still thankful, though, for the time we had. There were a lot of good times. We took the kids to a lot of places. We'd go to pumpkin patches during Halloween, egg hunts during Easter, you know, little things that you just did. We spent a lot of time with her family because she had a big family. We were always doing family things for Easter, Christmas, Thanksgiving.

We would also go on trips. We would go to Orlando frequently to see her family down there. We have been to Disney World several times. We would go to the Ozarks, just doing a lot of special things that I always wanted to do as a family.

As the kids got older, Julie would go to every select volleyball tournament with Annie and I would go to Jimmy's select baseball tournaments. Most of the time those were on the same weekends. When Jimmy decided he didn't want to play select baseball, I was able to go with Julie to Annie's tournaments. Those were good times. We had a lot of fun with the other families.

Julie had a fair amount of friends who may have been single or divorced. My friends, for the most part, were married and had families. My friends accepted her, but I don't think she felt as comfortable with my friends. I would be going to functions by myself, and Julie would do something else. It just snowballed as we got older.

Before we had kids, I remember bringing Julie down to Florida to see where I lived, where I played, and meet some of my friends. Those were special times. We had been through so much together and she was there for me every day. For me, being as sick as I was, to have so much support was phenomenal. I would tell her every day that I loved her more that day than the day I married her.

She was supportive to that point. However, when I got sick and needed to be on kidney dialysis three times a week, I was pretty much on my own. There were some very difficult days I had to get through. Like when I would get gout. It's just an incredible pain, like you're literally moaning and moaning. Julie had already moved out, and it wasn't like she could do anything, but it's just that you wanted someone there.

I remember one day falling out of my bed and hitting my head on the wood floor. I was really dazed. I tried to get a hold of Julie and couldn't. Finally, I did talk to her and she said she couldn't get home to help me. I actually remember calling a dad from Annie's volleyball team and asking him to come over. I crawled to the front door and unlocked it when he came over to help me.

I got served with papers the week of my birthday, February of 2019. My birthday was on a Monday, Feb. 25. She sent me a note wishing me a happy birthday, and then she served me with papers the same week. That was kind of odd.

The divorce wasn't final until December of 2020. It's just very sad. I still love Julie. I believe that we were good for each other. I'm not going to say my illness wasn't hard on her. She went through many rounds of me being sick. I'm sure it was hard. I was always hopeful that we could work things out, but it just didn't happen.

Chapter 17

A Difficult Summer

I'll never forget the summer of 2018. I was in my third year of kidney dialysis and I knew I needed a heart and kidney transplant soon. I was separated from Julie, and I had a hard time with that. And then there was my good friend Dominic Barczewski.

Every year Dom and his family would go on vacation to Florida. They would stay down there quite a bit, maybe three or four weeks a year. This time — I think it was July of 2018 — Dom was driving back to St. Louis with his son and his son's friend. They were just outside Huntsville, Alabama when they stopped at a gas station. Dom was filling the gas tank and I think Dom's son and the other young man were inside getting a snack or something. When they came out, Dom was slouched over on the car.

Fortunately, they were at a gas station and not driving. Immediately, they called 9-1-1. As it turned out, he had a very serious stroke. It just so happens the largest stroke center in Alabama is in Huntsville, so they were able to get Dom to the center quickly, which I'm sure had a great deal to do with saving his life because it was a severe stroke. We learned later that there were doctors in St. Louis who could not believe he was alive. They read his medical records and thought Dom looked much better than the records indicated.

Dom's wife, Annette, made plans to get a medevac plane to bring Dom home to St. Louis. They had him stabilized and, before you knew it, he was back in St. Louis at Barnes. At that point, he was in ICU, so no one was getting in to see him. But he started making slow progress. Within weeks, he was over at the rehab center, which is part of the Barnes complex.

The doctors at Barnes were amazed at how he was recovering. I remember going to see him one day and he was sopping wet with sweat because he had been working out so hard. But he was having a problem with seizures. He was taking a lot of medication to prevent the seizures, but it seemed like they kept coming. He would have a good week and then get a seizure, and that would set him back.

"We've Got a Heart For You"

Dom kept up with the rehab. He got out of the hospital and came back home. It was not long after that I finally got called for my transplant. It was a Saturday in August. I just had dialysis that morning and I was at home sleeping. Apparently, everyone was trying to reach me, but I wasn't answering the phone until Julie called and said a nurse was trying to reach me. I told her I wasn't sure I wanted to do this. Then I talked to the Barczewskis and they came over.

At that point, Dom wasn't good with leaving the house very much because he was still having a fair amount of seizures and wasn't feeling all that well. But, when I talked to him, Dom and his wife were at my house within 15 minutes. Dom is just telling me in his broken speech, "Tietj, you gotta go, you gotta go. You gotta do this. Jim, you gotta get out of bed."

One of the nurses called me from the hospital and said, "we've got a heart for you." I said give me 30 minutes to think about it. She was kind of shocked at my response, but I was half asleep. I guess calmer minds prevailed and I got myself ready. I quickly packed a bag and we were on our way to the hospital. I got down there probably around 4 or 5 o'clock.

I was fairly calm because I had been through this before. Nothing could start until the doctors checked the heart and made sure it was ready. So the night started to drag on. It was about 1 in the morning. Mike Redohl was in my room with Dan Flynn, who was the CEO of the U.S. Soccer Federation. Dan was a recent recipient of a heart transplant and we had become friends. Mike McCartney, another friend I grew up with and worked with at A-B, was there, too.

Dr. Masood, my surgeon who honestly didn't look over 25, came into the room and started going over everything that could happen. I told him, "Doc, I've been through this before. I don't need to hear about it. It's just going to put a little fear in me, so let's don't go through all this stuff." So Mike Redohl, being who he is, wants all the details. Mike started unloading questions on him, like "How many of these have you done successfully?"

The doctor was kind of dodging the question. I started to believe that this was his first, so I told Mike to shut up. I told him let's assume this is his first, but he knows what he's doing. Let's just get this done.

Dr. Masood explained that this was going to be a hard surgery because of scar tissue from the first transplant. He said, "I'll have to cut out that scar tissue. Most likely we're not going to be able to close you up right away. I'll have to keep you open with an ice pack in there."

Right before they took me down, I had an unsettling episode in the room. One of the nurses came to get me and take me down, but I wasn't ready to go because I had not said all my goodbyes to my friends. It could have been the last time I saw them alive, and they meant a lot to me. It got emotional. I jumped out of bed, got in her face and told her I'm not going down now. I told her, "I need to say goodbye to my friends. I love these people. Just go out and I'll let you know when I'm ready."

It actually got worse. I heard her talking in the hall to someone about me, and I just erupted. I flew out into the hall and told the nurse on the floor to get her out of my sight and I don't want her on this floor right now. I don't want to see her. She's not taking me down. They acted quickly. I was on edge, but these were people that meant so much to me and had been with me through my first transplant, they were there when I went through my Stage 4 lymphoma.

They couldn't do the surgery without me, so we were going to do it when I was ready. I got down to the operating room and the doctors and nurses had heard about what happened upstairs. I just said, "Hey, it's over. I don't need to talk to anyone about it. That's behind us. It's time for me to focus. Let's go."

The surgery itself went pretty well. The kidney went in first, then the heart. The heart started right up and it went exactly as Dr. Masood said — he left the ice in there. When I came to, the first 36 hours were decent, but apparently I had what was described as C Dif (*Clostridium Difficile Infection*) and pneumonia. I knew something wasn't right because they weren't closing me up when I thought they would. The doctor would come in and say, "Jim, your heart and kidney are functioning very well. Just hang in there. Keep fighting."

I knew he wasn't going to lie to me, so if he's telling me I can do this, I knew I could. But it was hard. They had me on some heavy meds and I was unconscious a

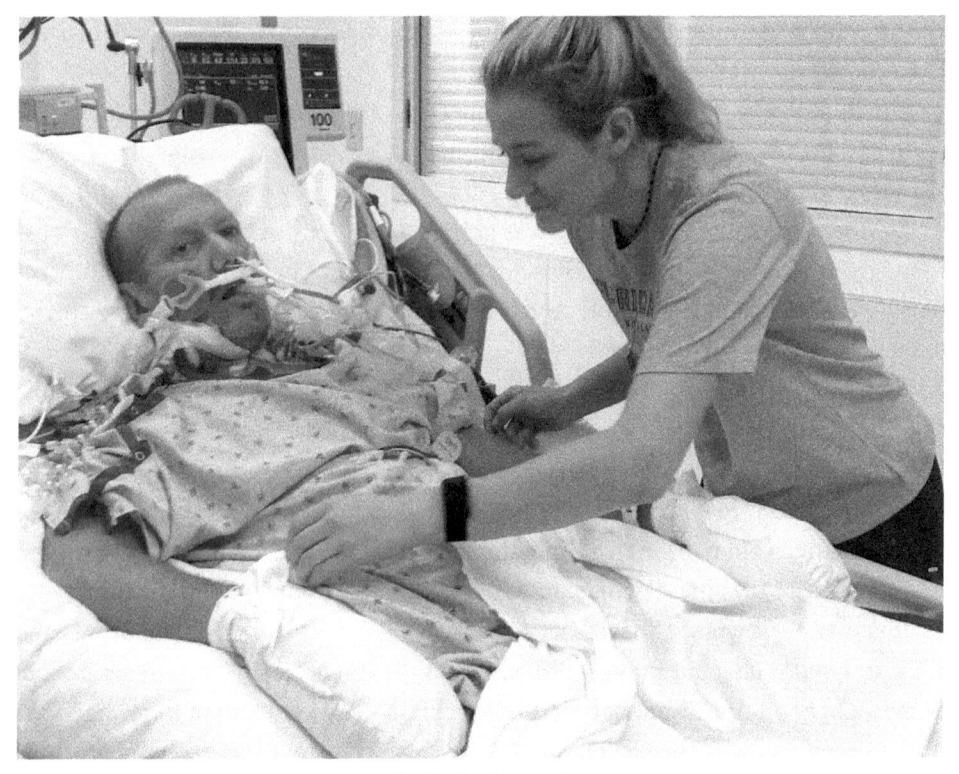

Jim in the hospital

lot. I was having terrible nightmares… about my wife, about my daughter. I felt like there were evil things in the room.

They ended up wrapping my hands in gauze, big giant balls like a boxer's hands because I didn't trust any of the doctors besides Dr. Masood and my nurse. There was a guy who came in and represented evil to me. His badge looked a little different to me, and I took my hands with all my might and pushed him away, so they had to wrap up my hands.

A Rough Recovery

There was about a 48-hour period where I could have gone either way. They started weaning me off the meds and I slowly came back to life. I was in the ICU for almost 10 days. It was hard. I couldn't get any rest. Doctors and my nurse were constantly in there. I thought if I could go to a step-down floor and get some rest and therapy, I could get much stronger. Since my vitals were great, I was able to talk them into it.

So as they saw the symptoms for C Dif and pneumonia go away, they thought that would be a good idea.

Within 24 to 36 hours, the therapists began coming in. The first day of therapy was not easy. I would be sitting in this tall chair — I'm standing, but I'm strapped to it — and it's holding me up. I'm just sort of moving my legs. Once I started it, I would do it on my own. But I had a great therapist. She worked me so hard every day. We did both physical and occupational therapy.

I was in a cardiac step-down for another 15 days maybe. Just to get my strength back was not easy. I never had any idea it would be this difficult. I guess it was a combination of my age (*58 at the time*) and being hit with pneumonia and C Dif. But I pushed myself pretty hard. In the workout room there were small steps you had to climb, certain things you had to do in the stairwell. I just took it as a personal challenge.

There was another challenge I didn't expect. Because the breathing tube was in my mouth for so long, when they finally got the tube out of my mouth, I couldn't speak for over 10 days. Dr. Masood kept saying he was confident my voice would come back, but I was a little concerned about my vocal cords being paralyzed. All of a sudden one day it started getting better.

In addition to great doctors, nurses and therapists, I had so much support from my friends. Like Kurt Billmeyer, a guy I grew up with and played with in high school. Kurt was probably the toughest guy on our team. If you wanted someone to be in front of you in a fight, Kurt was the guy. But one night when I was in the hospital, we were having chicken parm. They had to cut up my food because my vocal cords were swollen, so Kurt is in there cutting up my chicken piece by piece and feeding it to me. It made me feel good that he would do that for me.

I didn't realize this at the time, but Bill Colletta came to see me when I was in the hospital. After I got out, his son's fiance said to me, "Jim, Bill was in your room when you were unconscious — and he held your hand." When I heard this, I just teared up. Bill was in my room and held my hand for an hour. That's the kind of friends I have.

Mike Redohl was there just about every day. Mike and his wife, Liz, would sometimes show up between 5:30 and 6:30 in the morning, and they would always be working the nurses. They always brought donuts or cupcakes, something to give to the nurses to make sure they were taking good care of me.

Gary Ullo was there every day. He would be gently hitting on the nurses in one way or another. There were even times I was fading in and out of consciousness and I could hear him flirting with the nurses. One time I said softly, "Gus, give it up, will ya?"

Mike McCartney, who is a lawyer, was sort of my legal counsel while I was in the hospital. Since my wife and I were separated, I really wasn't sure what was going to happen. Mike was in on every doctor's meeting, even though they had no idea who this guy was. He was taking notes and he would explain everything to the family and friends about what was going on.

When you think of my guys, they all played a role. Kurt never told anyone what he did. Bill never told anyone he was there holding my hand. Mike Redohl doesn't tell people how much he was there. McCartney, Gus... they were all just there. At that time, I had a lot going on, my marriage, my health. They all just showed me unconditional love.

Before the hospital released me, they wanted me to see the doctor that did the cancer surgery on my neck. I hadn't seen him since my surgeries. He looked at my vocal cords and said, "Jim, they're not paralyzed. You're going to be fine."

At that point, it was time to go home. Julie picked me up and drove me home. Gary had a friend from St. Margaret Mary who came over the next day and ran some errands for me. I had a cane, but that night I decided I'm starting on my own. I threw the cane in the basement.

I got in my car the next morning, drove myself to the Workout Company and walked in the door. I have an idea of how hard I can push myself. The doctors would have had a cow if they knew I drove myself and that I went to the gym. They didn't want me driving for two weeks, but this has worked for me. This was the beginning and every day I got stronger.

Chapter 18

Meeting My Donor's Family

It was late November or early December of 2018 when I decided to write a letter to someone in my donor's family. I wasn't sure who because I had to go through Mid-America Transplant to do that, so I was not able to connect to them directly. I thought since we were approaching the holidays and some time had gone by since my transplant, maybe this family would be happy to hear that there has been some good out of this. With the holidays coming up — their first holiday without their son — I knew that they would not be in great spirits.

I just wrote, "Here's my life, here's my family's life, how my father and sister died, here's how this has helped me and my family. I believe that if your son or daughter could have selected someone to donate to, they would have been proud to have selected me." It was just a very carefully written letter to make sure I wasn't going to offend anyone. I was just showing gratitude.

So the holidays went by, January went by, February went by, and then mid to late March I received a letter from a female who said she was my donor's mother. She said her name is Cheryl Ellis. It wasn't a real long letter. She said she started the letter many times but was never able to finish it. She said she would like to stay in touch with me, but she wanted it to be gradual because it was hard for her to do.

I responded to her with more gratitude, just saying that she should do whatever she felt was right for her. I received one or two more letters. We ended up exchanging

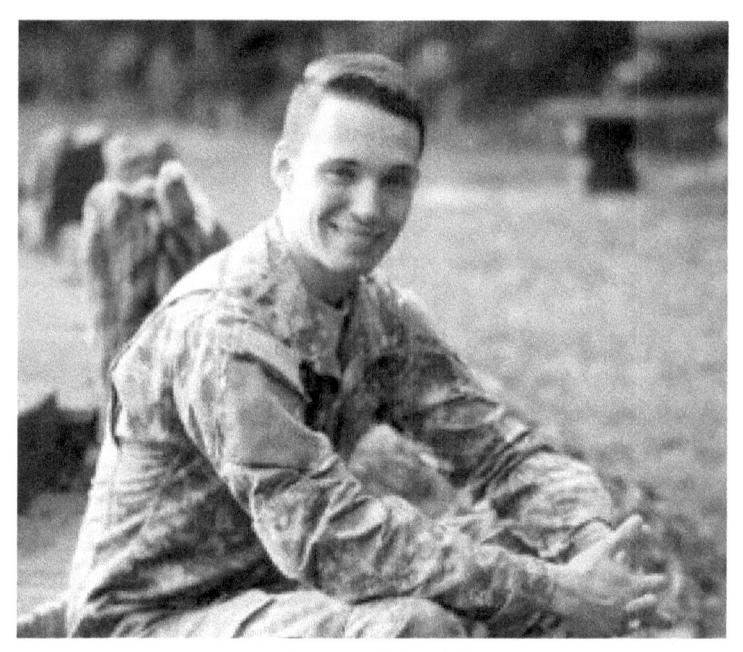

Jim's donor Colton Ellis

email addresses and started communicating via email. Since I had her name, I would see some of her posts on facebook. I could tell it was still very difficult for her.

I remember one day getting a letter from Cheryl. I took it to my bedroom and I started to open it. I always thought the heart I got was from a female donor because the weekend of my transplant there were two drowning incidents that happened in St. Louis on the Meramec River. So, as I opened the letter, a picture fell out and hit the ground in front of me. I looked down and saw a very young man with his young son, and I just collapsed on the bed behind me. I put my head in my hands and thought, "Oh no, not someone like this."

I picked the picture up off the floor and started reading the letter. Cheryl's son was an only child. I read a little about Colton, that he was 23 and his son Carson was 2. Colton was a combat medic in the Missouri National Guard. She raised him by herself. Obviously, they were very close.

I would send her notes to let her know that I was thinking about her. I would tell her how I was doing, that things were going well. I told her a little about my family's story, hoping that she would think they did the right thing by donating Colton's organs. I know she had many bad days — every day had to be tough. If I can say something to put a smile on her face for a few minutes, that would be good for me.

Meeting At Mid-America

At this point, we decided to meet. We were already talking to each other and we felt comfortable enough to talk to each other in person. She made plans to come up to St. Louis in July of that year so we could visit. We were trying to decide on a place where everyone would be comfortable for us to meet, so we decided to meet at Mid-America Transplant.

Mid-America let us use their offices. They asked if they could record the meeting and take some pictures. I said it was fine with me, but I asked them to contact Cheryl and see if it was OK with her. So they got very much involved in our meeting.

I told Cheryl at any point that if she changes her mind, it's fine with me. I didn't want to put any pressure on her. I didn't want her to feel forced into anything. So, she came up to St. Louis with two of Colton's best friends. One was in the National Guard; the other friend was a paramedic in Cape Girardeau, where they were from.

Cheryl and the guys arrived first and they took them to a section in the back area. I arrived second and they put me in a meeting room. I had brought her a few gifts, a rosary and a mass card, and a few other really small things. They had brought a really nice book with pictures of Colton throughout his life. They also had t-shirts made and had these metal wristbands with a message printed on them.

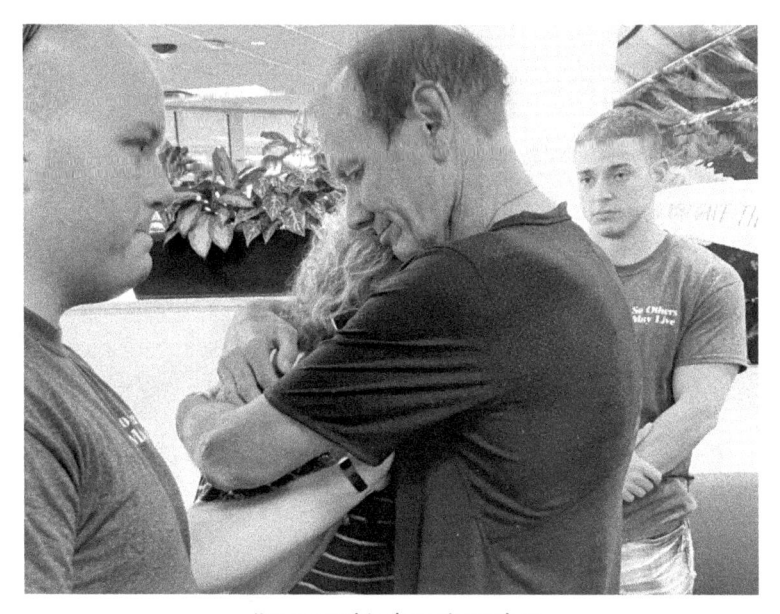

Jim meets his donor's mother

The motto of the combat medics in the National Guard is "We Serve So Others May Live." To me, it was incredibly powerful because even in his death, Colton chose to serve others like me, serving so others can live.

So it was time to meet. I could see her from the beginning of my walk. I could see the two friends. I didn't take my eyes off her the whole time we walked towards each other. I got to her and immediately — there was no introduction — I put my arms around her. She put her arms around me and we embraced for a long time. It was an amazing moment for both of us. Not a lot was spoken, but I think that made the moment even more powerful. I just whispered in her ear, "I promise there is nothing I will ever do to damage this heart." His two friends joined in and we all hugged together.

One of the ladies from Mid-America Transplant had a stethoscope. Cheryl and the two friends were able to hear Colton's heart. I was pretty skinny at the time, so you could really hear the heart beating strong. When she was listening to it, she was literally in tears. She had her head on my chest. It was an amazing moment. While obviously heartbroken, I believe that she was happy with who got the heart. On the way home, she sent me a note and said that Colton's friends felt that his heart was in a good place.

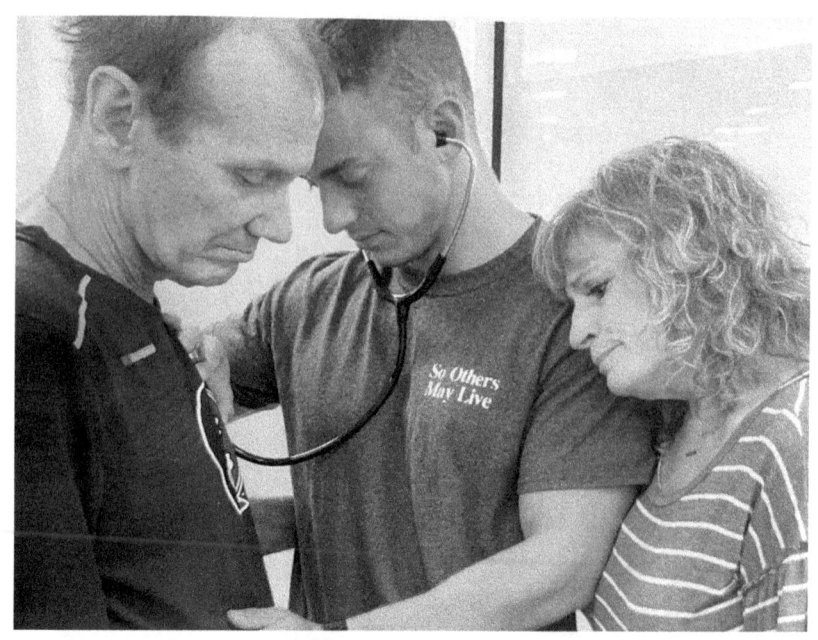

Jim with his donor's mom, friends

We met again the following spring when she came up to visit her brother in Kirkwood. I had my granddaughter Gia with me and she and Colton's son Carson hit it off right away. They were running around playing. We sat down and had lunch on the patio. It was a nice little gathering.

Another Meeting

We had discussed going down to Cape Girardeau on the anniversary of Colton's passing. Cheryl told me she would like me to be there, so in August of 2021 I drove down there in the morning and met them at the cemetery. I met several of Colton's friends. I was trying to understand my role there, but I think they felt good about meeting me.

I think about Cheryl a lot. We have a unique relationship. I feel like I can pick up the phone and call her, and I think she feels the same. I have two amazing organs from her son. Once I got through rehab and started going to the gym again, I thought I was doing something special. But, no, it has to be him. His heart is amazing. My previous ejection fraction on my old heart was in the mid 50s, which is mid to low normal. With Colton's heart, my ejection fraction has always been between 67 and 70, which are numbers I had never seen in my first 26 years of having a transplanted heart.

Cheryl knows all about my health problems. I continue to let her know how the heart and kidney are doing. I assure her that I am taking care of them and that I would never do anything to damage them. I am so grateful for her son's sacrifice.

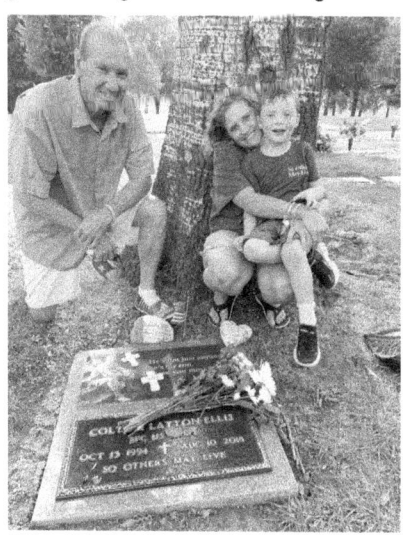

Jim at his donor's grave

Chapter 19

Mid-America Transplant

My relationship with Mid-America Transplant is well over 30 years now. My first role with them post-transplant was going with them to different hospitals throughout Missouri, sometimes talking to nurses, sometimes talking to families about transplantation. I would go to them as an example of how transplantation has affected me and try to educate them, allowing them to hear first-hand from someone who has had a transplant.

As a procurement agency, Mid-America Transplant does everything there. They have people who go out across the state to speak to families to let them know about the great things that can happen for other people during the worst time of these people's lives. Their role is to talk to the family and promote being a donor. Can you imagine having that discussion when someone has just lost her 23-year old son, and he's your only son? But that's where it starts.

Not only are they doing that, they're working with local hospitals to keep organs viable until they're ready for transplantation. Sometimes they will bring the potential donor to St. Louis or they will go out and harvest the organ on location. When they get to Mid-America Transplant, they have about seven ICU rooms where they take care of patients and multiple cath labs where they do a bunch of tests. Within 30 minutes, they can get the results to the doctors at Barnes. It allows much more work to be done at Mid-America so when the doctors are ready to go, the organ is sent over to Barnes. All they have to do is get the patient opened up and do the transplant.

My sister Laura had her heart transplant in 2001. After her transplant, she went to work for Mid-America Transplant. She did a lot of guest lectures at high schools throughout the St. Louis area. After my second transplant, I reached out to Mid-America and said I really want to help. I want to be part of it. I don't mind talking to people. Wherever you see a fit or need, I want to be that guy. So I've talked to multiple high school groups or early college groups of students who want to go into the medical field. I've spent a lot of time doing that.

Mid-America and Barnes know all about our family history. Laura's daughter Kortney has been transplanted twice. Fortunately, we have all had the same transplant team. Cindy has been our coordinator forever.

Sharing My Story

One of the coolest things I did was when Dr. Masood asked me to come to a learning program at Barnes one weekend. They had doctors from all the hospitals in St. Louis and some outside of St. Louis on stage reviewing different cases. All the hospitals were sharing their success stories, the best guys at St. Luke's, the best at Mercy, the best at Barnes, and so on.

The presentations were not specifically about heart transplants, but it was more about heart disease and things you could do before you get to the

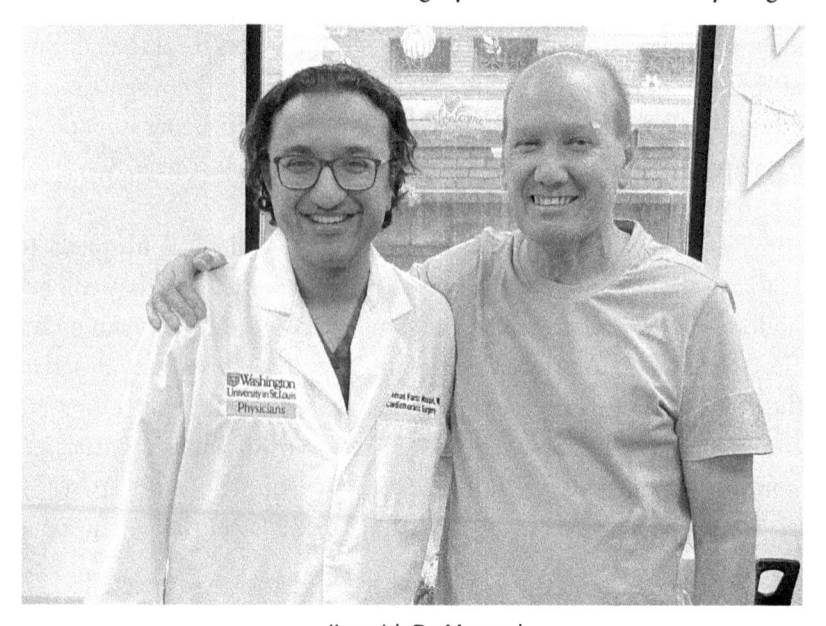

Jim with Dr. Masood

transplantation stage. It's all about keeping people alive by alternative methods. It was really interesting.

They had a big audience there. Some of the nurses in the audience were people who had taken care of me. Some of them knew me very well.

The thing was wrapping up and Dr. Masood started texting administrators in the back of the auditorium where I was sitting. He wanted them to ask me if I wanted to come up on stage and speak. So, he introduced me, I spoke and told my story. I tried not to make it all about me. I talked about the nurses. I was just trying to talk about the overall success story. It was all about the team — it's the nurses, the doctors, the technicians, the people at Mid-America, myself. I call it the "Chain of Life."

When I was finally done, I was floating. I was pretty happy that I had the chance to talk. I guess I'm proud of my accomplishments, right? So, I'm going back up the stairs and I'm looking down because I didn't want to trip and embarrass myself. I didn't realize it until I got to the top of the stairs, but everyone was standing and clapping for me. I guess it's because they're getting to see a success story that they don't always see. It was just one of the coolest moments I've ever experienced.

The Chain of Life

To me, the Chain of Life really starts when someone decides to be a donor. And Mid-America Transplant is one of the strongest links in this chain. Without them, a transplant isn't going to happen. There's just so many people that are involved, and they do this every day. They're just so amazing at it.

Then you've got a team that takes care of patients after a transplant. For example, I had C-Diff. I had pneumonia. Fortunately, I had a post-transplant team that took care of me. There are just so many people that have to be on their game every day. If one link in the chain fails, it might not have a good outcome.

I meet these people and it's like I'm in the presence of rock stars. When we were younger we thought professional athletes were great, right? No, my rock stars are the people from Mid-America Transplant. I think about the doctors and nurses. When you're in ICU 24 hours a day, it's that nurse that I always want in my sight. He or she is my rock star.

For information on organ donation, visit the website for Mid-America Transplant at midamericatransplant.org.

Chapter 20

Pneumonia

Because our immune system is shut down, transplant patients are very susceptible to pneumonia. I don't think I've ever met a transplant patient who hasn't had pneumonia. I've had it at least 12 times.

When I get pneumonia, I know the exact moment when it's time for me to drive to the hospital. I've done it with St. Louis U. I've done it with Barnes. I've done it with St. Anthony's (*now Mercy South*). Just about every time I've driven in there, the doctors tell me that I did the right thing.

There are two incidents of pneumonia that I remember most. One was when I learned that I was getting a lifetime achievement award from St. Louis U. They were recognizing me for all the trials and tribulations I went through. Joe Clarke, who was the head soccer coach at SLU at the time, said they were going to officially present me with this really nice crystal soccer ball at a ceremony for me.

Unfortunately, I got pneumonia and had to go to the hospital. There was something in the newspaper that week about the recognition, so I got a call at the hospital from an older gentleman who said he was a buddy of my father. And he had another guy who was a buddy of my dad. They read about me getting the award and asked if they could come see me in the hospital. I told them that would be great.

It was a pretty cool moment. In fact, I was in tears. Never have I talked to someone who really knew my dad. They were able to tell me things about him. They said he was an athlete, an engineer, a hard worker, an outdoorsman who loved to fish. I even think one of the guys played basketball with my dad.

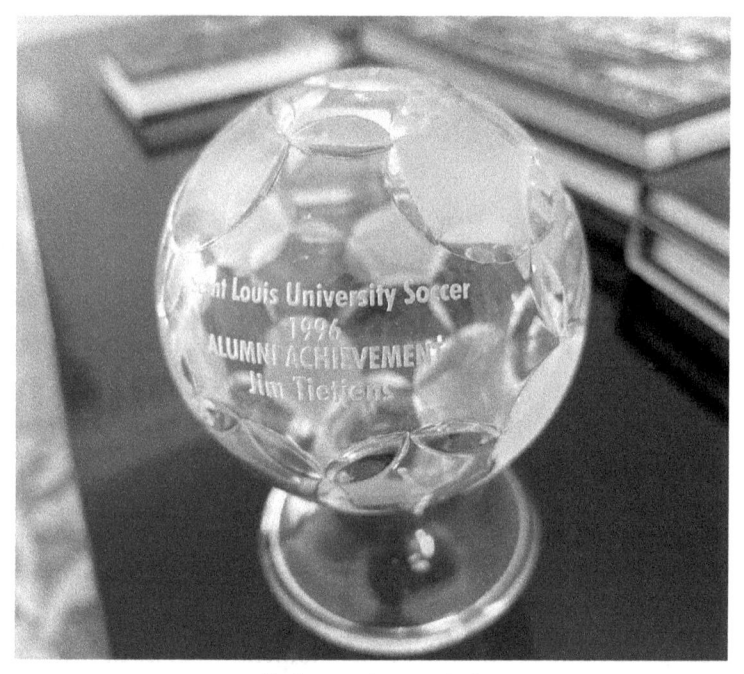

Jim's crystal soccer ball

I asked them if they would go down to St. Louis U. and accept the award for me. They said they would be pleased to do that. So I called Joe Clarke and told him that I'm sorry that I can't get down there, but I have these two gentlemen who knew my dad and they would like to accept the award for me. And that's what they did. I let Joe know when I got out of the hospital that I appreciated the honor.

A Really Bad Experience

The other incident I remember came when I had to go to St. Anthony's. We had just had our soccer reunion for the '76 championship team at Crusoe's Restaurant in Oakville, and during the reunion I could tell I was getting sick. And it was bad. So I drove myself home, took a shower and tried to get in bed. But I knew I had to go to the hospital. I was so sick I couldn't get out of bed. I had the chills. I finally willed myself out of bed and drove myself to the hospital.

This was during the time when I was on kidney dialysis, and it was a really bad experience. I got there at like 9 or 10 at night and I was there until the next morning. They put me in a satellite emergency room — I guess it was an overflow thing. It was so cold in there. I couldn't talk. I was trying to call people to help me, but they just kept me there. I'm going to call it like it is — they just forgot about me. I kept trying to tell them that I was freezing. They didn't give me blankets. I got sheets. Even when I told them I'm a transplant, they just ignored me.

When I got up to the floor, I was much worse. My blood oxygen level was very low, so they put a mask on me really tight. I kept pulling the mask off. I was really upset because I'm trying to reason with the doctor. He's telling me to keep the mask on and that I could die. I told him I know I need to keep the mask on, but it's too tight. I said you have to give me something to sedate me… please!

Finally, they did give me something. As soon as they did, I was OK. Later that day, I found out that my daughter Annie flew back to St. Louis from Florida. I see Annie come into the room and I look over at Julie, like what's going on? Julie told me that the hospital told her that she needed to bring my daughter home. They knew there was a chance I could die.

St. Anthony's wanted me out of that hospital, so they sent me over to Barnes. I got down to Barnes and they said they had to set me straight. They quickly got it under control. I had too much fluid in me. They just tried to get me stable so I could get back home and continue with my dialysis sessions.

St. Anthony's had never let me down until that day. I never paid the bill. There was a co-payment due and I called them to tell them the bill isn't getting paid. I explained everything to the collection agency and they said that they understand.

They never bothered me again.

Chapter 21

My Oakville Brothers

I loved every second of my time playing on youth national and professional teams. But nothing compares to the relationships we began to build when I joined my high school team in 1975. We were teammates and best friends back then. We're so far beyond that right now — we're like brothers.

We did the stupid things kids did when we were younger, but we all came from blue-collar families. We all believed in hard work. We all had strong faiths. And now it's a brotherhood. We all share this unconditional love for each other. It's just there. You know it's there. No matter what happens to you in your life, no matter who it is, you know that any of the other guys are going to be there for you. It's the best thing in my life.

Captain Gary

When we won the state championship in '76, Gary Ullo was the captain and leader of our team. Everyone worked hard, but Gary worked harder than anyone else. When there was running, Gary was always the first guy to finish. I tried so hard to beat him, but I never could.

Gary is someone I respect so much. I think we're both on the same page faith-wise, and that has helped us stay close over the years. He loved hockey, so we spent time going to hockey games. If there was a big soccer game in town, we would go watch those games together. When our club coach went into the hall of fame, it was myself, Dom, Gary and Bill Colletta who drove together to see Mr. (*Don*) Bayer get inducted into the St. Louis Soccer Hall of Fame.

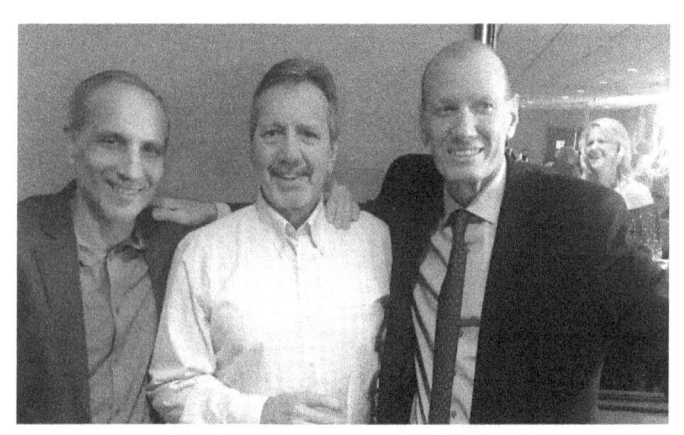

Jim with Gary Ullo and Kurt Billmeyer

The fact that Gary has organized anniversaries and get-togethers is not surprising. Gary sells advertising for the Archdiocese of St. Louis and one of his customers is Cardinal Glennon Children's Hospital. He came up with the idea to host reunions of the '76 championship team and raise money for the hospital. We've had over 12 reunions and we've raised over $20,000.

That's not a huge amount of money, but this is a small group of guys. We had about 19 guys on our roster back then. Unfortunately, some have passed away. If we get 10 or 12 guys at the reunion, that's a lot. In January of 2022, I think we got well over $2,000. In 2023, we raised over $4,000. It's the most we've ever raised. Our goal each year is to get at least $1,976 in honor of our '76 team.

The Backfield

Our backfield on that '76 team — Dominic Barczewski, Bill Colletta, Kurt Billmeyer and Roger Schallom — was special. Those guys took me under their wing and gave me confidence. They helped me a great deal.

Bill Colletta is the nicest guy you would ever want to meet. But I'll tell you what. When he got on the soccer field, he turned into a different guy. He was so intense and so focused. He just battled.

Kurt Billmeyer was the funniest guy in the world. No matter what anyone said, he had a funny line for everything. He was pretty quiet on the field, but Kurt was never going to run away from a fray. No one ever intimidated him.

Roger Schallom was very tough physically. He was not the most skillful player, but he played his position very well. He knew how to push his man out wide where the least danger was. He just played tight man-to-man defense and never backed down against anyone.

Our strength was our backline, and Roger was a big part of that. He just focused on his responsibility. If everyone did that, we knew we would be successful. That's why the defense worked so well. Everyone just did their role.

And then there was…

Dominic

Dominic Barczewski could have played anywhere in the country. He went to UMSL (*University of Missouri-St. Louis*) and became a two-time All-American. After college, he was drafted into the North American Soccer League by the New York Cosmos, the most famous professional soccer team in America at the time.

Dom was known for his ability in the air, but he had this touch for a big strong defender that was really amazing. It was so good that he would win the ball, then take steps with it to get the ball out of danger. That's why he went so far. Dom was always smooth, quiet, intense, physical. No one was more physical than Dom. He would never go into a game afraid of who he was facing.

After our pro careers, Dom and I remained close. He was with me the night I met Julie. After we were both married, we would hang out a lot because our kids were the exact same age. My daughter Annie is the same age as Dominic's son and my son Jimmy is the same age as Dominic's daughter.

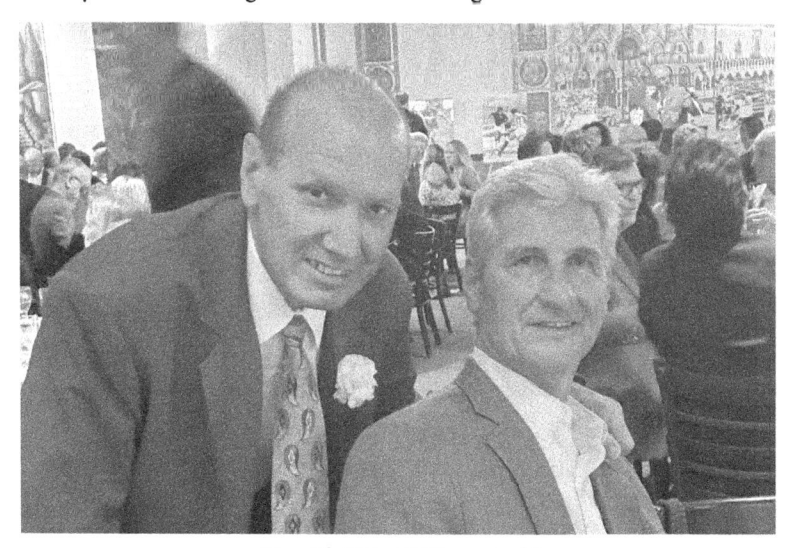

Jim with Dominic Barczewski

We would take trips together. I remember one time we went to the Lake of the Ozarks and stayed at a friend's house. It was Bob Lattinville, the lawyer at Rawlings, and his lake house was called the Lattin Villa. It had everything you ever wanted. We would open the refrigerator and it was filled with kids drinks and adult drinks.

One day we went down to the boat area where they had two jet skis. But the jet skis didn't work. Between myself and Dominic, neither one of us could fix anything. But I'll be damned. The two of us got those jet skis running. We had the kids on the back with life jackets on. We had a flippin' ball.

Dom has always been there for me. When I had my first heart transplant, he was at the hospital almost every day. The day before my second transplant, Dom and his wife came to my house to get me out of bed and help me get to the hospital. He had just had his stroke that summer and was not comfortable going to someone's house. When he came over the house I was touched. I was inspired.

That's why I've always tried to be there for Dom. After his stroke, he was making slow progress, but his wife Annette was reaching out to medical professionals at area hospitals to find a solution for his seizures. No one seemed to have the answer. Quite possibly, the answer didn't exist.

Off To Germany

Annette researched around the globe and found this doctor in Germany by the name of Nils Thoennissen — we called him Dr. T — who was working with the Cord Blood Institute of Munich. She made contact with him, talking to him weekly, and after a while she was buying into what he was doing. He believed he could improve Dom's condition by using this cord blood.

So Annette and Dom planned a trip to Germany to see Dr. T. I decided I didn't want them to go by themselves. I was so worried about something happening to Dom, a seizure on the plane, a seizure on the streets. I didn't want Annette to be by herself if something like that happened. That was my concern.

I hadn't been there in years, but I was comfortable in Munich. So we ended up going to Munich in the fall of '19. When we landed at the airport, our ride didn't show up. I just thought, worst case, we would hop in a cab and go to the hotel because we were staying at a Courtyard by Marriott.

So we jumped in a cab and the driver is driving about 120 miles an hour. Annette is on her iPad calculating the kilometers into miles per hour. As he's going faster, she's looking at me, going "Tietj, Tietj, we're at 130 miles an hour." It was a

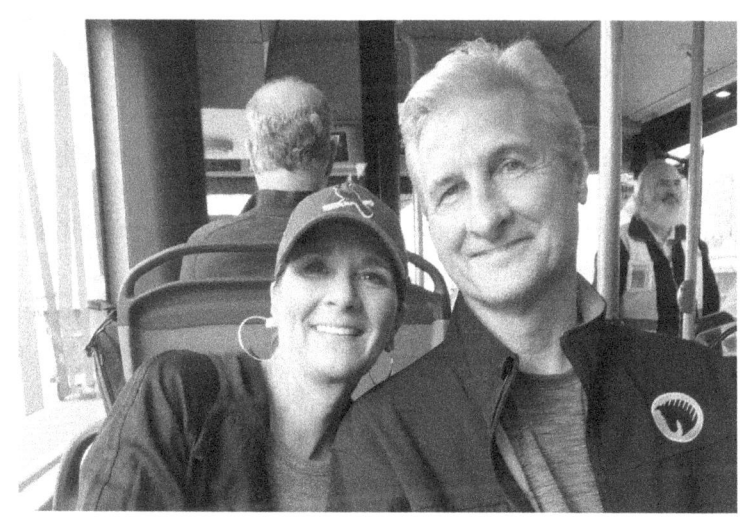

Dom with his wife Annette

little scary. Finally, I asked the driver to take it down a few notches. We're here for medical treatment and we want to make sure we get where we're going in one piece.

Fortunately, we got to the hotel safely and checked in. We got a hold of Dr. T. He said he would come meet us after work, so he came to visit us at the hotel. We hit it off right off the bat. You could tell that he was a genuine guy. We went into a restaurant, had something to eat, and started talking soccer. We didn't talk much about anything medical. By the end of the night, he said that he would come and get us the next day and explain everything about the treatments for Dom.

The third day we were there we went into his office for Dom's first treatment. The doctor explained that when the cord blood gets into your body, it's able to go right to where the illness is. Dom ended up having three or four treatments and was feeling well. He had no seizures while we were there. I don't think Dom has had any seizures since.

Time For Sightseeing

We had a great time in Germany. We did another thing that was kind of a dream come true for me and Dom. We went to Allianz Arena, where Bayern Munich plays their home games. The tour is really cool because you get to go into the locker rooms. We went into Bayern's locker room and all the jerseys were hanging up, and then we went into a separate locker room for the German national team.

Then we went on the field. For Dom and me, we were like kids in a candy store. We were always jetting off on our own, the tour director calling us back because we were going to places where maybe we shouldn't be. We were acting like, "We can't understand you, we're Americans." By the end of the day, we told them that I was friends with Gerd Muller and Dom had played with Franz Beckenbauer. They probably thought we were crazy, but we didn't mind. It was an amazing trip.

If you ask Dom and Annette today if the trip was worthwhile, they would say absolutely. Is Dom 100 percent? He's not. But his mind is as sharp as can be. He's been an inspiration to me. He's had to fight through a lot. I've been faced with things that can be healed. I think we kind of inspire each other.

Chapter 22

Peripheral Artery Disease

While I was on the trip with Annette and Dominic in Germany, I remember we walked up a mountain Dominic's doctor wanted us to see. As we were walking up that mountain, my calves were really burning. It didn't feel right. There was nothing wrong with my wind. It was just my calves. I suspected something was wrong there.

On the last day we were in Germany, I was cutting my toenails and I actually cut some skin on my small toe. That was the night before we were leaving, and it really hurt. We got back to St. Louis and it wouldn't heal, so I went to see a podiatrist at St. Anthony's. I told her I was doing a lot of walking on the street since the gym was shut down because of COVID, and the walking was making my toe hurt more and more.

So the podiatrist sent me to St. Anthony's to get a Doplar study to take a look at the blood flow in my legs. At this time, it wasn't good at all. After probably nine months, she was finally able to get the toe healed. It's the first wound I had. Later during that summer of 2020, I got another wound on my fourth toe, right next to my little toe. That one happened when I was power washing my house and I was wearing sandals. Water got between the sandals and the skin and created a blister.

The blister turned into a sore, but it would not heal. It actually got worse. It scabbed over and then the scab turned black. It was black for several months and I decided to see a surgeon down at Barnes, a vascular surgeon. He looked at it and asked if I wanted him to try and peel the scab. He started peeling and it was incredible pain. He immediately turned around to his nurse and said we have to schedule — he used some language to describe it as "number four toe, right foot, amputation…"

I heard the word amputation and I thought, "O my God, no…" He said there's a good chance that if we didn't take the toe off right away, an infection could form and go all the way up my leg and he would have to take the leg off, so he amputated the toe. At the same time, he did a procedure to try and open the blood flow to the foot. There was about 30 percent blood flow going to that foot, but it already had signs of gangrene, so he took the toe off.

More Circulation Difficulties

I have what is called peripheral artery disease (*at its worst, it's known as Chronic Limb Threatening Ischemia*), a severe condition that limits blood flow to your limbs. It's a disease that can affect people who have had organ transplants, especially kidney transplants. When I was first checked, two of my arteries were completely blocked and the third was semi blocked. I had about 25 percent blood flow into my feet and you need at least 30 percent to heal a wound. If you don't have circulation, you can't heal. I've had cuts in the past that take a long time to heal.

I have had wounds on both feet. I don't know how that happens. I think sometimes toes get dry in the winter time and sometimes the skin splits and cracks. I wash my feet every night and coat each foot with vaseline. I also use betadine to keep it clean and prevent infection, then put a sock over the foot to keep the treatment on it and prevent skin from cracking.

My doctor — Dr. Patrick Geraghty — has done a handful of surgeries on me. Since there is one main artery from the waist to the knee, they would go into my groin area and put in a couple of stents. I had some blockage there.

Because of this lack of blood flow, I have had nearly a dozen procedures to open the blood flow to my feet. The arteries are so thin and hard to work on that they generally don't stay open for a long time. No one has created a process to work on these arteries that is foolproof. My doctor's goal has been to save my limbs. If a wound doesn't heal, we have to look at other options, which could be amputation.

Chapter 23

Hall of Fame

I remember the night I got a call from Jim Leeker, president of the St. Louis Soccer Hall of Fame. There was a whole lot going on that night. My daughter Annie was in a car accident, and I had been on the phone trying to find out what was going on with her. She was in the hospital with a concussion.

The call came in pretty late, sometime between 9:30 and 10. I asked Jim if I could call him back because my daughter was in an accident. I finally got back to him. It was probably 10, maybe 10:30, when he told me that I had been selected for the hall of fame and he wanted to be the first to tell me.

I had become friends with Jim because I was the guy letting everyone know how Dominic was doing after his stroke in 2018. Dominic was going into the hall of fame that November, and I was there the night he was inducted. I was in a mask, post-transplant. At that ceremony, Jim mentioned that I was in the house that night — and pretty much everyone in the St. Louis soccer community knew about my health challenges. He made a comment about working to get me in the hall of fame and most of the people there stood up and applauded. That was nice of Jim to recognize me.

When I called Jim back and he gave me the good news, obviously, I was happy. It wasn't a goal of mine to get into the hall of fame. It's obviously nice to be recognized, but it's not something you spend a lot of time thinking about. There's a lot of great players in the hall of fame, there's a lot of great coaches, and a lot of great people who have contributed to soccer who are in the hall of fame. It's a nice family to be a part of.

I was happy to share the news with my son and daughter, Julie and my friends. I called Mike Redohl, Dom and Annette, Gus, Kurt, Bill, Roger. I also talked to Johnny Hayes and Tommy Groark. Johnny and I were roommates on the national team and in college, and Tommy was a teammate of mine with the Fort Lauderdale Sun. I called them because I knew they were supportive, and I knew they would be happy.

I was supposed to be inducted in 2020, but the event was canceled because of COVID. After a year's delay, they held the dinner at Rose of the Hill, the banquet hall for Favazza's Restaurant. It was a great night. I had three tables there for family and friends, many of them representing Oakville — seniors from our state championship team, and some of the underclassmen.

Sonya Bayer, Don Bayer's widow, was there. A buddy from A-B, Jeff Esserman, was there. My good friend Mike Redohl and Mike's dad, who has been an incredible mentor in my life, were there, too. As for family, Jimmy, Annie and my sister Laura were there. Julie was not there, but she watched the live stream.

A Big Speech

There were 11 inductees in the Class of 2020. I was one of the last guys to go because they went in alphabetical order. The highlight of my speech was not about wins and losses, or keeping the ball out of the goal. It's more about the friends, the brothers that you meet along the way and keep with you afterwards. I was blessed to play on teams on the southside and the northside team that went to Scotland. I was blessed to play at St. Louis U. I felt like I was a part of the family right there in that room.

Jimmy is rarely sort of moved emotionally to anything, but when I was done with my speech, he stood up and gave me this unbelievable bear hug. He told me he loved me and was proud of me. That meant a lot.

Annie's reaction was a little different. As I was waiting for my turn to speak, I was checking my notes. She kept interrupting me. "Dad, can I have some of your chicken?" That's how Annie is, but I'm sure she was proud of me. After the speeches, we took a great picture of the three of us together.

What I remember most from that night is that the people who have been most important in my life were there to share that moment with me. They were as much a part of my success as I was, maybe more. There were so many people to celebrate with. All the people I grew up with were there. My grade school coach (Mr. Fitz) was invited, but he had dialysis treatment that day and couldn't go. I'm not big on

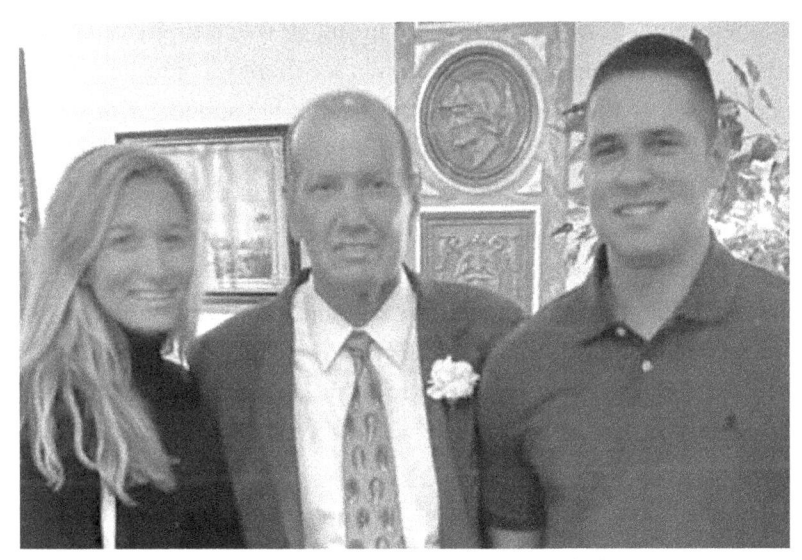

Jim with Annie and Jimmy at the St. Louis Soccer Hall of Fame banquet

celebration, but I'm as happy as can be when all my friends are there to share the moment with me.

Two people I wish could have been there were Mr. Bayer, who had passed away, and Jim Bokern, my high school coach. Jim wasn't in town. I really would have loved to have had him there.

I really wanted to go out and have a few beers after the ceremony. Dominic had a rough night, so he and Annette went home. The Billmeyers went home, and so did most of the others that were there. I hadn't been out in ages because of the COVID thing.

It was just a special night. After you get in and are able to celebrate, you want the night to continue. It's like when you win a championship. You don't want to leave the locker room because you just want to take in the moment as long as you can. I've done that a couple times in my life. That's what I've done when I've been on a championship team, just sitting in the locker room and taking it in.

A Night to Remember

The soccer family in St. Louis is so big and so close. The hall of fame dinner is the one event where you see so many people from that community, some of the people who were your idols growing up. I remember seeing Al Trost there. At one time, he was considered the best player in America. It was very cool to see him there.

I had other interactions with guys who meant so much to my career, like Dave Brcic and Larry Hulcer. Just to be able to embrace them was special. Larry told me how proud he was of me. Larry has always been a big supporter of mine while I was going through my health challenges. He was a teammate of Dominic's with the Cosmos before he was traded to the L.A. Aztecs. He got rookie of the year playing for the Aztecs as a defensive midfielder. As for Dave, I knew him from the U.S. Olympic team. We were on multiple trips together.

On the way home from the induction ceremony, I talked to Julie. She said I set the record for the longest speech. I think my speech was about 16 minutes; it was supposed to be about five minutes. Trust me, Jim Leeker was sitting over there and I was getting the eye. But the speech was well received. Most of the people stood up and applauded.

Julie's father always wanted the chance to see something like the hall of fame dinner, but he did not have a chance to go to the banquet because he was in an independent living place. We took some pictures of me with my green hall of fame jacket to show him that I was there.

When you get a green jacket, it's pretty cool. My biggest concern was that I had lost so much weight from my surgery that my jacket would not fit. Fortunately, it fit perfectly. Same thing with my ring. My fingers were skinny when I was measured, but that fits, too. Wearing the ring and jacket was a cool thing. I'll wear them when I go back to the next dinner.

Now that I'm in the hall of fame, it's up to me to start pulling for some of my high school teammates. There's no doubt in my mind that Kurt Billmeyer, Bill Colletta and Gary Ullo should be in the soccer hall of fame. No disrespect to anyone who is in the hall of fame. They're all great players. But if they're in there, Kurt, Bill and Gary belong there, too.

Chapter 24

My Sister Laura

My story would not be complete if I didn't mention a few things about my sister Laura. She worked in the Mehlville School District for 21 years, mainly as a kindergarten teacher. I became aware of Laura's need for a heart transplant in 2000. I had not talked to her in quite some time, but I felt it was critical to reach out to her and let her know what it's like to go through a transplant. I had already been transplanted for eight years, and I wanted her to see that my life was pretty good.

Laura had her heart transplant in 2001 (*she was in the hospital on 9/11*). After her transplant, she became involved with Mid-America Transplant and committed herself to the promotion of organ donation. Since she had been a teacher, she developed training protocols and did presentations where she would talk to people about organ donation. She wrote a curriculum for St. Louis University so doctors could go through the whole process of following someone from death to being a donor. She did guest lectures in almost every school district in the St. Louis area. She became knowledgeable and well respected within Mid-America Transplant.

As Laura got older, she started to have kidney problems, which is not a surprise to transplants. After about 20 years, her kidneys were bad and her health started going downhill. Her heart was still in good condition, but she needed a new kidney. Unfortunately, she had complications with the kidney transplant, along with viruses and then at some point COVID. She also had some cancers, so she was dealing with a lot. A combination of things beat her down and she was never able to regain her strength and fully recover. Laura passed away in March of 2023.

What's amazing is I never heard her complain one time about her health. Even about four weeks before she passed, we were talking about the next Christmas holiday and how to plan it. She knew there was a good chance she wouldn't be alive for the next holidays, but she knew that the holidays were a tough time for me. She was still thinking of me.

Over the last 20 years, we became very close. We never made a big deal about our health challenges. I still remember her saying, "We just deal with it. The doctors told us what to do, we did it, and that was it."

That attitude is what we grew up with. You'll never hear us being sorry for ourselves. It just isn't in us.

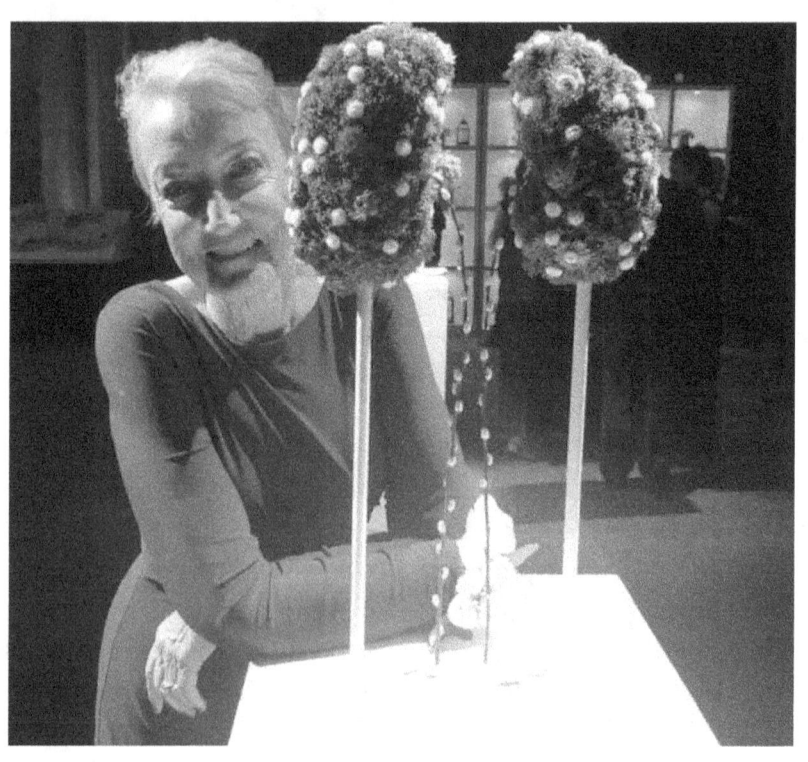

Jim's sister Laura

Chapter 25

Thanks / Acknowledgments

There are many health challenges that I have overcome in my life, but do I really think I could have done that on my own? I'm kidding myself if I believe that. It wasn't just me. I needed God's help. Divine intervention has made a big difference in my life.

I've had a lot of suffering, but God and Jesus and Mary have given me the strength to endure that suffering. They've given me special friends to support me with that suffering. They gave me some of the greatest medical people in the United States. All these people in one way or another have become friends, too. They have put wonderful people in my life, people to lift me up when I need to be lifted up. They're always there when I need them.

To some extent, I've been lucky. Actually, I feel like I'm the luckiest man in the world. If you sit back and take a deep look at it, I have two children and a granddaughter who don't have the bad heart gene. I couldn't complain to God one bit about what he has given me to handle. Fortunately, he has given me strong shoulders and strong friends, and I have been able to rely on them.

I have so much to be thankful for. I thank God each day for the many blessings in my life. And some of those blessings are these people who have helped me endure my health challenges:

JoAnn Richter (my mother) — Everything I've accomplished and who I am today is because of my mom and her strength and what she taught me. My mom taught me that we can overcome anything, and that belief has always been with me.

You will never hear us feeling sorry for ourselves. It just isn't in us. It is what it is. And that comes from my mom. She passed away in 2016. The night she died I told her that I will be OK because she has taught me everything I need to know.

Jimmy and Annie — Jimmy and Annie were 7 and 5 when my health challenges began. What drove me was my dream to be a father, and knowing that I was able to achieve that, I had a huge responsibility to raise them. They have grown up watching me face my health challenges, knowing that "Dad would get better." I am so proud of both of them for what they have been able to accomplish.

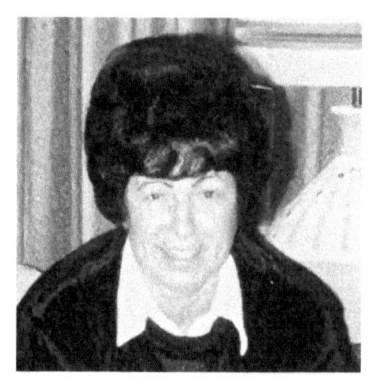

Jim's mother

Julie — During the first transplant, Julie was always there for me. She never wavered. She knew I would get there, and that was a good feeling. She never doubted me, which gave me confidence. She was the same during my struggle with cancer, too.

My sisters Karen and Laura — Karen fought her battle quietly and alone and she passed alone. I wish I would have been at her side to hold her hand and I wish I could have carried her cross. Laura fought so hard for over two decades and we became very close. I never once heard her complain. It was not uncommon for her to get a major curveball every year and she always accepted it all with so much grace.

Harold Richter (my step dad) — Harold had a blue collar job at Southern Equipment Company. He worked a lot of nights and just never took the time to attend my games or be a part of that. But I appreciate what he did coming into our family and taking us on. Harold apologized to me on his death bed for not being there for me. I told him I accepted his apology, that I loved him. He was a good man with a wonderful heart. And the Richters always made us feel part of the family. They were amazing.

Mike Redohl — Mike pretty much put his life on hold when I was sick. He and his wife Liz would show up at the hospital as early as 5:30 in the morning to make sure the nurses were OK. Mike always believed in bribing the nurses. There's nothing like a donut or a bagel that says, "This is a special person. Take care of this person." Mike made me a priority in his life. He knows I struggle at times. I get lonely. He calls every day, usually in the morning because he wants to make sure I'm up and moving. I know why he does it. I value it. I appreciate it. And I need it.

My teammates — My teammates accepted me and gave me confidence when I was in high school, and they have continued that support through the years. Just think about the things they have done for me — Dom and Annette coming to my house the day before my second transplant, Bill Colletta holding my hand while I was unconscious in the hospital, Kurt Billmeyer cutting up my food and feeding me as I was trying to recover, Gary Ullo organizing the reunions and helping us raise money for charity.

Mike McCartney — Mike, a lawyer who now runs his own business as a financial advisor, is another guy from the neighborhood I grew up with. I also worked with him at A-B. While I was in the hospital for my last transplant, he was sort of my legal counsel. Mike was in on every doctor's meeting. They had no idea who he was, but he was taking notes and then explaining everything to family and friends about what was going on with me.

Coaches — Mr. Fitzgerald (*grade school*), Mr. Bayer (*club ball*), and Jim Bokern (*high school*). They gave me the opportunity to play and built up my confidence.

Dr. Craig Reiss — When I got sick the first time, he sent the police out looking for me. I was having episodes, and at any time these episodes could have ended my life. It wasn't easy to find me, but he did. Then that one day in the hospital when they all came running down the hall to check on me, that was the scariest moment of my life. I told Dr. Reiss that I just want to be a father. He assured me that I would.

Dr. Muhammad Masood — There was a point after my second transplant when I was sick in the hospital with C-Diff and pneumonia and I just thought to myself that I can't do this anymore. But I kept hearing Dr. Masood's voice, "Jim, you can do this. Keep fighting." Dr. Masood saved me, in more ways than one. He just told me my heart and kidney were doing great. If he's telling me that, then I'm going to believe him.

Cindy Pasque (nurse coordinator) — She has been my transplant coordinator since my first transplant and we have become very good friends over the years. Honestly, she's still my transplant coordinator as well as coordinator for my sister's daughter. She's really been a mentor, a friend and just someone I can always lean on and talk to anytime.

My entire medical family at Barnes Hospital — This is a larger family that includes surgeons, the heart team, the cancer teams, the vascular team, the kidney team. It was the nurse team that was with me 24/7, the techs, the people that delivered our meals, those that cleaned my rooms and those that often had to clean me. My PT people were amazing, the ICU teams, the cath teams. There are so many that I have missed. Thank you for allowing me into your family even when I may not have been worthy of it. Thank you for holding my hand and making a difference.

Both my donors — I never met the family of my first heart donor but know the donor was very young. This was an amazing heart that beat true and strong for over two decades. I would challenge this heart every day and every day it showed me just how strong it was. And then came Colton Ellis, who was a combat medic in the Missouri National Guard. Colton was a Christian who was loved by so many. Even in his passing, Colton chose to save others. In addition to me, Colton was able to save or enhance the lives of many donor recipients. He was a true American Hero.

Cheryl Ellis (mother of Jim's heart/kidney donor) — Back in July of 2019 I had the honor and privilege to meet my heart and kidney donor's mother, Cheryl Layton Ellis. Cheryl lives in Cape Girardeau as did her son Colton (*my donor*). Getting to meet a donor's family member is never a given and is something I consider to be a sacred honor. Every time I talk to Cheryl I learn more about Colton and the amazing son, father, grandson, husband and friend he was. On the day I met Cheryl I made a promise. I want to make Colton very proud of how I am living and how I am taking care of his amazing organs. Thank you, Cheryl — and Colton.

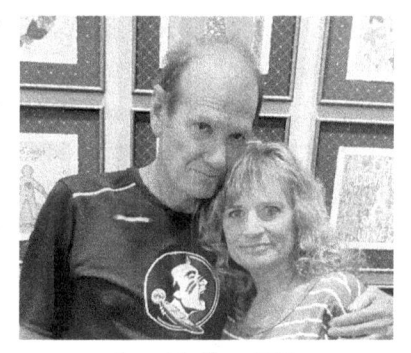

Jim with Cheryl Ellis

My father Jim — I hope you are able to look down and approve of how I am living my life. I look forward to the day when we can be reunited as a family and share a huge family hug. We might have to wait a while as this heart and kidney that Colton gifted to me has a lot of life left in them. By the way, dad. I wanted to thank you for your service to our great country. One last thing, pop. Just curious as to what you think of the white corvette? Maybe

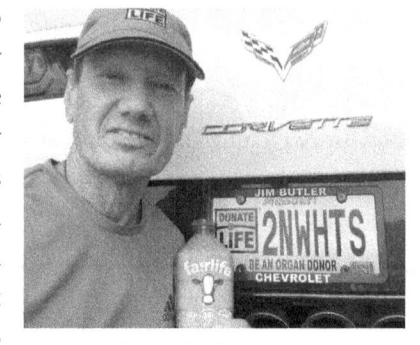

Jim with his corvette and personal license plate

send me a sign sometime that you approved. Colton is a car guy, so I am pretty sure he approves. If you have not done so yet, take the time to say hello to Colton. I am sure mom has already done that. Catch you on the other side, pops. Just be patient. I love you. Your Son, Jim.

Note: A special thanks to the following organizations for their assistance with photos: Barnes Hospital, Florida State University, Mid-America Transplant, Oakville High School, Rawlings Sporting Goods, St. Louis University, Washington University

More praise for Jim Tietjens

"I have distinct recollections of Jim before his first heart transplant. He had been a competitive athlete and was in the prime of his life with a young family prior to his diagnosis of heart failure. He knew that his condition was hereditary and he had witnessed the devastating impact of the cardiomyopathy on his family and friends. Jim faced his illness with courage and strength, even as his body began to weaken. There is no doubt that the same determination coupled with a wonderful and supportive family have allowed him to survive and thrive for 31 years. Jim represents a true success story in transplant medicine — it has not always been an easy journey, but I suspect he would tell us that it has been most fulfilling. I also know that he has a deep appreciation for the families of his donors who gave him the most precious gift imaginable." — **Dr. Joseph Rogers**, cardiologist, President and CEO Texas Heart Care Institute, heart transplant team

"Jim has lived his life following his heart transplant with gratitude and passion. Even when he needed a second heart transplant with a kidney transplant he remained positive and continued to exercise and work. He is a model transplant patient who has honored his donors by taking great care of himself and the organs he received. Jim also believes in giving back and consistently has been an advocate for the heart transplant community. So when I hear Jim's name, I just smile and say he's an amazing guy." — **Dr. Joel Schilling**, cardiologist, Washington University, heart transplant team

"Jim Tietjens is a lifetime Olympian. As he left the sporting realm and entered the heart patient world, Jim brought with him all the traits that allowed him to succeed in sports. When Jim came to us, his heart was about to fibrillate and stop functioning entirely. Jim knew this but had the presence of mind to create a plan that allowed him to stay alive until that miraculous day arrived. Once that day came, Jim adapted and brought a new game plan. The plan was simple, and he still carries out this plan today, 31 years later. Jim never allows himself to be a patient. I am so proud of him and honored to call him my friend." — **Dr. Craig Reiss**, cardiologist, St. Luke's Heart Health Specialists

"Jim is an athlete. His determination, motivation, and drive to get better was evident from the first day. Jim is wired to work hard to achieve his goals. Heart transplantation is no easy feat. Jim made recovery after heart transplantation look tremendously easy. He is a motivational speaker for our patients. His positive attitude and energy is inspirational to our patients, as well as the team of nurses, physicians and allied health practitioners. We, as health care professionals, are honored to be a part of his journey of transplantation." — **Dr. Muhammad Masood**, Professor of Surgery, Washington University, Jim's heart surgeon

"The first time I met Mr. Tietjens in the Nephrology clinic was a sense of amazement. Anyone who has an organ transplant, even without other problems, and survives and thrives for 20+ years cannot be but meticulous about everything, including his medical care. The second thing that struck me was "This is a hard nut to crack" and " the man is arrogant." However, the more I got to the real person, AKA Jim, the worry about arrogance changed to an admiration of his tenacity and his willingness to do whatever it takes to be better. He realizes, like many people with genetic family diseases, that his fight is not a fight for himself, rather for all his loved ones. To some degree, I think he was also fighting to make sure he honors all the nurses, staff and physicians who worked tirelessly to keep him alive. Mostly,

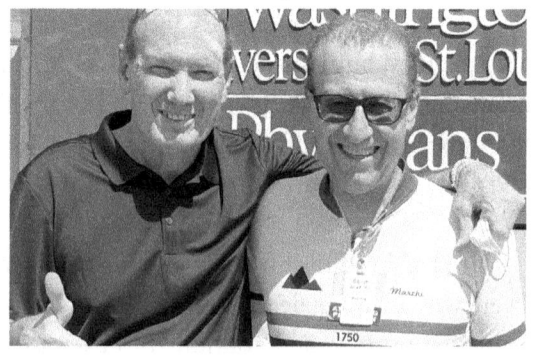

Jim with Dr. Jarad

his tenacity was to honor the legacy and the unbound generosity of the donors and their family. Trying to do anything less than perfect is not Jim's way." — **Dr. George Jarad**, Nephrologist, Washington University, Jim's kidney doctor

"Jim embodies resilience. He never let two cancers, two heart transplants and a kidney transplant define him. During his chemotherapy for Hodgkin lymphoma, he found a way to tuck away the anxiety and stress, and attend to his life — being present for his family and continuing to work full-time. Jim shows us all how to live optimistically, appreciate the present, and not dwell on adversity." — **Dr. Nancy L. Bartlett**, oncologist, Washington University, Moments Chair in Medical Oncology

"When I hear Jim's name, the word that comes to mind is persistence. For decades a cardiac diagnosis and its consequences has set the bounds of Jim's life. Jim has pushed those boundaries and always sought greater opportunities and better answers for himself and his family. Pushing back against 'too hard' or 'not now' or 'we don't know' has required remarkable persistence and I admire Jim for that." — **Dr. Justin Vadar**, cardiologist, Washington University, heart transplant team

"Jim Tietjens is a rare bird, perhaps my only patient with limb-threatening ischemia whom I had to beg to slow down! Jim presented with foot wounds caused by two common sequelae of diabetes: severe atherosclerosis of the arteries in his calves and feet, and loss of sensation in his feet from neuropathy. This is an unfortunately common and dangerous combination of diseases that carries a high risk of amputation. But unlike most of my patients, Jim was extremely diligent about exercising on a daily basis. He told me that maintaining his health was a way for him to show his gratitude to the donors of his transplanted organs. I really appreciated Jim's insight and commitment, although it took some time to convince him to take enough of a break to allow his wounds to heal. Jim simply never gives up, and always tries to give back. One way that he is giving back is by participating in studies of the patient experience of limb-threatening ischemia with the Vascular Cures Foundation. This time commitment

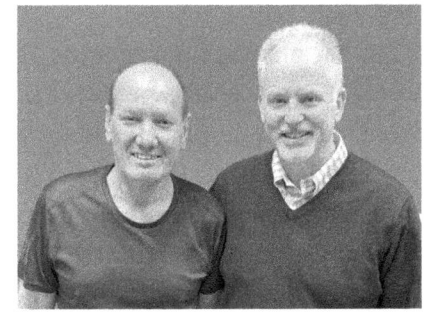

Jim with Dr. Geraghty

helps caregivers better understand the impact of this disease — and the various treatment options — on patients' quality of life. Jim understands the importance of both established and innovative treatments, and is always fully engaged in the shared decision making of how we treat his complex disease state. He is a genuine trailblazer, and it's been a privilege to be on his care team." — **Dr. Patrick Geraghty**, vascular surgeon, Vascular Surgery, Washington University

"I feel very fortunate that I have a relationship with Colton's heart and kidney recipient. When Jim first reached out I knew I wanted to meet him and hear Colton's heart beat again. But it was still extremely hard to not be resentful and bitter that my son was gone and someone else had his heart. It took me a while to get to the point that I was mentally and emotionally ready to have a relationship with Jim. But I am so happy that I do. Jim is the most gracious, thankful, and kind person. Anytime he has met any of Colton's friends he makes sure to let me know how grateful he is and what good care he takes of Colton's organs. Jim reaches out regularly to check on me and let me know he is thinking about Colton. I am proud of my son for making the choice to be a donor and saving lives." — **Cheryl Ellis**, mother of Jim's heart and kidney donor

"When I think of Jim, no thought ever comes to me without the words strength, resiliency, courage and 'never give up' also flashing through my mind. Taking a moment to actually reflect on the myriad of challenges he has faced and continues to face, both physically and mentally throughout his life, it's truly amazing what he has and continues to accomplish. He is an inspiration and example to me when I face challenges of my own, a reminder you can overcome even the greatest obstacles." — **Kurt Billmeyer**, high school teammate

"As the athletic trainer of the Fort Lauderdale Strikers, I had the privilege of having this new goalkeeper move in with me at my townhouse, The Lofts. Jim was quiet and the one we could always count on to look after the group if we had a long night out at our Pierce Street Annex post game parties; I always knew I would make it home safe! This is the guy if I had a daughter I would want as her husband. Always respected others first, but his love for his car — don't think it was ever dirty — his love for working out and enjoying Fort Lauderdale and the beach. Jim always treated my family like they were his. Jim is competitive, realistic, passionate for others, and it's an honor to have crossed paths and spend quality time in the sun with my pal." — **Eddie Rodger**, former athletic trainer, Fort Lauderdale Strikers

"I've known Jim since his high school days at Oakville where he led his team to a State Championship. College, international and professional soccer followed. Every step was a proving ground to test his willpower — and he met every step head on. His life certainly had more than the usual setbacks. He faced every one with the intensity he applied to stopping shots as a goalkeeper." — **Terry Michler**, Hall of Fame soccer coach, CBC High School

Foundation to Advance Vascular Cures

Chronic Limb-threatening Ischemia (*CLTI*) is an advanced stage of Peripheral Artery Disease (*PAD*). PAD affects 8-12 million Americans and is often unheard of until diagnosis. About 2-5% of patients with PAD will develop CLTI, which is the final stage of PAD that can lead to amputation of toes, feet, or legs.

Understanding CLTI begins with ischemia, which is a severe condition in which there is not enough blood flow and oxygen to a part of the body. Without blood, cells and tissues begin to die, causing damage to parts of the body. A narrowing or blockage of an artery usually causes it. Signs and symptoms of ischemia depend on how quickly the blood flow is interrupted and where it occurs. This condition won't improve on its own and requires medical attention by a vascular surgeon or vascular specialist.

You can learn more about ischemia and CLTI from information provided by the Foundation to Advance Vascular Cures, a non-profit dedicated to improving vascular health through research and education: https://www.vascularcures.org/s/VC_Focus_Ischemia_FINAL-HR.pdf. Here are some educational resources for patients: https://storage.googleapis.com/patient-toolkit/index.html#/ and for providers: https://www.vascularcures.org/pad-cad-virtual-learning-hub

The rates of PAD and CLTI are increasing due to a number of factors:
- aging US population
- smoking
- increases in conditions such as type II diabetes and obesity

PAD affects minoritized populations more than others, due to a number of factors such as lack of access to nutritious foods and/or quality healthcare. PAD may be the first sign of cardiovascular disease, and is a marker for increased risk for heart attack and stroke. Studies have demonstrated that PAD and CLTI are underdiagnosed and undertreated. CLTI is not something that develops overnight, and can't be reversed as easily as other conditions.

The major goals in treating PAD and/or CLTI are to improve limb outcomes and reduce cardiovascular "events" (*e.g., heart attack or stroke*), as well as improve patient quality of life. Some lifestyle changes you can make include a healthier diet and increased exercise, including walking and non-walking alternatives, such as cycling. Medical options include using certain medications, surgery, and endovascular treatment.

It is critical to speak with your healthcare provider about the best treatment option, as the risks of not taking action are high: amputation and mortality are real and far too common outcomes with CLTI. The Foundation to Advance Vascular Cures has a Patients are Partners program that connects patients, offers resources, and helps patients engage in research to eliminate the disease: https://www.vascularcures.org/our-programs/patients-are-partners.

Focus on Ischemia flyer

Patient Engagement in Research Toolkit

Peripheral Artery Disease / Coronary Artery Disease HUB

Patients Are Partners

Dr. Michael Conte, E.J. Wylie Chair, Professor and Chief, Division of Vascular and Endovascular Surgery, Co-Director, Heart and Vascular Center, Co-Director, UCSF Center for Limb Preservation and Diabetic Foot, is the Chief Medical Officer at the Foundation to Advance Vascular Cures, and a world recognized specialist in CLTI. Isabel Bjork, the CEO of the Foundation to Advance Vascular Cures, has a background in policy and regulatory reform and is dedicated to ensuring that research benefits patients directly and health inequities are reduced.

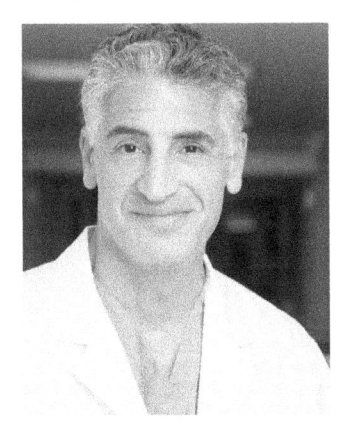

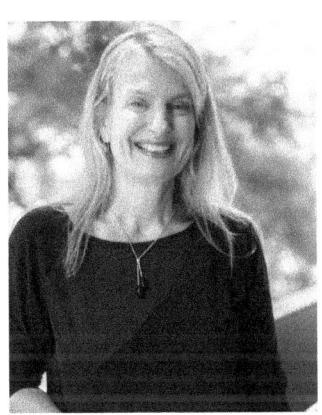

Dr. Michael Conte   Isabel Bjork

About the Authors

Jim Tietjens has an impressive resume as a soccer goalkeeper — state champion in high school, All-American in college, a member of the U.S. national team, and a professional keeper who won a championship with the Fort Lauderdale Sun of the United Soccer League. Following his playing career, he enjoyed success in the sporting goods industry as well as sports marketing. He underwent his first heart transplant in 1992. In 2018, he had a kidney transplant along with a second heart transplant. To this day, Jim continues to be an advocate for organ donation. Already a member of the St. Louis Soccer and St. Louis University Halls of Fame, Jim was inducted into the Mehlville School District Hall of Fame in 2023. He still lives in Oakville, Missouri and has two children — Jimmy and Annie.

Jeff Kuchno has spent his career working in the media and education fields. He has worked 27 years as a high school journalism instructor, retiring as a full-time educator in 2021. Prior to teaching, he served as the sports information director at the University of Missouri-St. Louis, where he received 13 national awards for excellence in publications. He is now a freelance writer and educator living in St. Louis. He and his wife Laurie have three children — Kevin, Bryan and Kristin.

Jeff Kuchno and Jim Tietjens share a passion for sports, fitness and exercise. They met in 2015 at the Workout Company in Oakville, and they have been friends since.

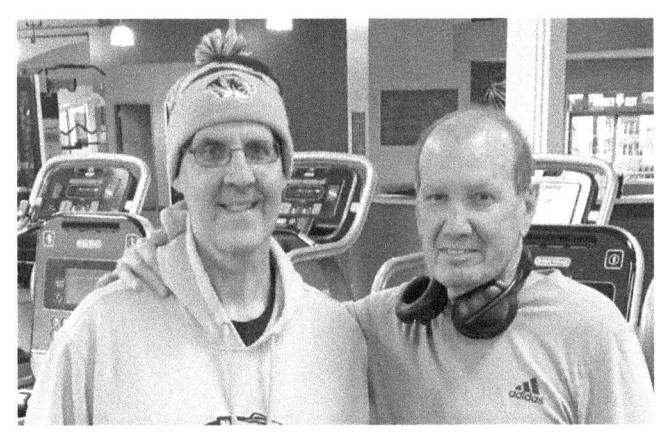

Jeff Kuchno and Jim Tietjens

Printed in the USA
CPSIA information can be obtained
at www.ICGtesting.com
CBHW071352300724
12434CB00003B/77